The Complete Guide to Cosmetic Facial Surgery

The Complete Guide to Cosmetic Facial Surgery

John A. McCurdy, Jr., M.D., F.A.C.S.

Frederick Fell Publishers, Inc.
New York, New York

Library of Congress Catalog Card Number: 80-70945
International Standard Book Number: 0-8119-0331-1

For information address:

Frederick Fell Publishers, Inc.
386 Park Avenue South
New York, New York 10016

MANUFACTURED IN THE UNITED STATES OF AMERICA
1 2 3 4 5 6 7 8 9 0

Preface

Cosmetic surgery is one of the more glamorized medical specialties and an area of considerable public interest. In the past several years, a number of books for the layman have offered a broad overview of cosmetic surgery. None of these volumes, however, has provided detailed insight into the history of the various operations; explained the procedures by which surgeons evaluate and select their patients; and included complete descriptions of the operative procedures, their limitations, and their possible complications. This is information which an increasingly sophisticated public desires.

The Complete Guide to Cosmetic Facial Surgery is an attempt to fill that void. Of particular importance are the sections recommending how to choose a competent surgeon and describing the qualifications of surgeons in the various specialties involving cosmetic facial surgery. The liberal use of illustrations and photographs is intended to enhance understanding of the text.

The reader should understand that the opinions and techniques of surgeons performing cosmetic procedures vary considerably. I have attempted to discuss the most common variations currently in vogue and to avoid passing judgment on the relative value of each. Every surgeon is the product of his past training and experience, and thus individual surgeons commonly employ different approaches to similar problems.

Acknowledgements

Dr. Keith Marshall, a Honolulu Oral Surgeon provided useful suggestions as well as pre- and postoperative photographs for the chapter on Orthognathic Surgery.

I wish to express appreciation to Charles Matsuda and Michele Bodine for their efforts in illustrating much of the text.

Contents

The
Complete
Guide to
Cosmetic
Facial Surgery

1

An Introduction to Cosmetic Facial Surgery

The American Medical Association defines cosmetic surgery as any operative procedure designed to change a feature of the human body that would be considered to be within the range of normal variation for a person's age and ethnic background by an impartial observer. A casual glance at the facial features of any large group of people reveals that a tremendous individual variation exists in the size and shape of the nose, ears, chin, and other parts of the face. For reasons that are difficult to define (see chapter 2), certain features are considered more beautiful or handsome than others. Considerable cultural influence, of course, pervades such esthetic judgments, and so facial features that are greatly valued in one culture may not be held in high esteem in another.

Cosmetic facial surgery, then, is designed to reshape or remodel parts of the face that fall within normal limits yet detract from the overall appearance of the person who wants such surgery. As facial characteristics are constantly on display, a large percentage of the entire field of cosmetic surgery is directed toward modification of these features. Examples include altering the shape of the nose, correction of prominent ears, augmentation of weak or receding chins, and rejuvenation of the aging face.

According to the above definition of cosmetic surgery,

procedures performed to correct severe deformities (i.e., those that are outside the range of normal variation) resulting from birth defects, injury, or disease, do not fall within its scope. Such operations are more properly placed within the broad realm of plastic and reconstructive surgery. Cosmetic surgery is only a segment of that specialty.

As cosmetic surgery is always elective (i.e., it is not required to save life or the function of an important organ), candidates for such surgery must be in sufficiently good health that the operative procedure will pose no threat to their physical or mental well-being. While this requirement does not necessarily exclude people with such chronic disorders as diabetes, high blood pressure, previous cardiac abnormalities, etc., such candidates must demonstrate proof of satisfactory control of these problems prior to surgery.

Most cosmetic facial operations are performed under local anesthesia with appropriate sedation (the patient is not actually put to sleep), and so the risk of these procedures is extremely low. As an additional safeguard, the vital functions of the patient are closely monitored with special instruments during surgery.

A Brief History
of Cosmetic Facial Surgery

The explosion in demand and availability of cosmetic facial surgery in Western society during the past twenty-five years has been astounding. Before then, surgery performed solely for cosmetic reasons was held in disrepute, and surgeons who performed such procedures risked ostracism by the medical profession. Consequently, such operations were performed in seclusion under a veil of secrecy. Because of the inherent risk to the surgeon's reputation, information about these procedures was not published in the medical literature, retarding the growth and development of this kind of surgery. Fees were high, and cosmetic surgery was available only to the wealthy and socially elite.

Other forms of facial plastic surgery, however, were acceptable during this period. Methods for reconstructing injured noses were developed by ancient surgeons and were later improved by surgeons during the Middle Ages. Techniques for removing excess eyelid skin of those whose vision was impaired by this overhanging skin were developed in Europe during the early nineteenth century. The improvement in appearance that followed this operation was noted but considered incidental.

Modern techniques of cosmetic nasal surgery began to evolve in the late nineteenth century. The first attempts to rejuvenate the aging face with a "face-lift" are thought to have been made in the early twentieth century.

The devastating wounds sustained by some during World War I provided a stimulus for the rapid development of plastic and reconstructive surgery, and further advances in the techniques of this field were made during World War II. Improvements in pre- and postoperative care and control of infection with the newly developed antibiotic agents contributed significantly to the expansion of plastic surgery.

Modern Cosmetic Facial Surgery

With the gradual repudiation of the Victorian standards of self-sacrifice and their replacement by the contemporary youth-oriented society—in which a premium is placed on the fulfillment of the needs and desires of the individual—the stage was set for the application of the improved techniques of plastic surgery to the area of cosmetic surgery. The accelerating public interest and demand for such procedures has stimulated improvement and refinement of cosmetic procedures and techniques. This demand, coupled with the trend towards subspecialization in contemporary medical practice, has encouraged other surgeons to join the traditional general plastic surgeon in the field of cosmetic surgery. These surgeons, specializing in surgical treatment of disorders of specific regions of the body, have acquired training and experience in cosmetic surgery of these regions and are called regional plastic surgeons. Among regional plastic surgeons active in cosmetic facial surgery are otolaryngologists, ophthalmologists, dermatologists, and oral surgeons (see chapter

4). Cosmetic surgery is currently one of the most widely publicized and glamorized areas of the medical profession.

Myths About Cosmetic Facial Surgery

In spite of an increasing medical awareness and sophisti-
cation in contemporary society, a certain mystique continues
to surround the cosmetic surgeon and his craft. Several myths
pervade society's conception of cosmetic surgery. The first is
that plastic surgery involves the use of plastic or other materials that are implanted into the body. While such materials
are used in some types of cosmetic surgery, most cosmetic
facial procedures involve altering facial structures without
using foreign material.

A second misconception is that the cosmetic surgeon can
remodel a specific facial feature to meet the exact specifications of the patient. This is certainly not the case, and this
myth is probably responsible for much patient dissatisfaction
with cosmetic surgery. As in most forms of creative endeavor,
the skill of the surgeon (or artist) is limited by the material
with which he must work. Although the results of some procedures are startling and dramatic, the candidate for cosmetic
facial surgery must be cautioned that the goal of the operation
is improvement in appearance rather than absolute perfection.

A third myth is that these operations produce no scars. In
actuality, scars are a universal accompaniment of any incision
made through the skin, and so they are always present after
cosmetic facial surgery. Their visibility is minimized by meticulous surgical technique and by placing incisions in areas
where they will be naturally camouflaged. These areas include junctions of facial landmarks (such as where the ear
meets the face) and natural creases or wrinkles.

A fourth misconception is that the term "plastic surgeon"
means that the physician is competent in all phases of plastic
and reconstructive surgery. As in all skilled fields, a surgeon
is a product of his training and experience, and these factors
vary from person to person. Techniques of cosmetic facial
surgery can be mastered only by painstaking exposure to, and

familiarization with, these methods and may be acquired by both regional and general plastic surgeons. This concept is discussed in detail in chapter 4.

Reasons for Seeking Cosmetic Facial Surgery

It is generally assumed that vanity is the only reason people seek surgical correction of displeasing facial features. Certainly, the desire to improve one's appearance has been a human characteristic through all recorded history. Such vanity constitutes an important part of a person's self-image, which is of paramount importance to his outlook on life. It should be remembered that vanity is not an entirely intrinsic characteristic, but is strongly related to a person's conception of how others see him. Thus, to a large extent, it is a product of the social niche to which he belongs or aspires.

In contemporary society, a premium is placed on "looking good" and on a youthful appearance. The influence of this standard in our culture is reflected in a recent survey of attitudes toward various facial features. As many as 23 percent of women and 11 percent of men were dissatisfied with one or more of their features.

It would be remiss, however, to suggest that vanity is the only reason people seek cosmetic facial surgery. In many cases the motive is economic. In the high pressure atmosphere of modern business, people often feel that the prestigious assignments or promotions may go to someone who presents a better appearance. In spite of the adage that aging is associated with maturity and wisdom, aging executives, both male and female, may sense that a more youthful appearance will help them achieve their goals. An improved appearance may bolster sagging self-esteem and offer a person a new outlook on life. Such motivation is not restricted to the motion picture or television industry.

Young adults often feel that certain facial characteristics detract from their appearance, undermining the self-confidence that is important to social development and adjustment.

Such social considerations, if properly evaluated and documented, may be valid reasons for cosmetic facial surgery.

On occasion, the cosmetic facial surgeon is confronted with a person who is so ashamed and embarrassed by his appearance that significant psychological problems have developed that interfere with his daily life. Cosmetic surgery may save such people from a lifetime of emotional turmoil precipitated by the ridicule of others, whether real or imagined.

Selection of Candidates
for Cosmetic Surgery

The surgeon screens all prospective candidates for cosmetic facial surgery to insure to the best of his ability that the motives of these people are realistic and valid. One obvious requirement is that a facial deformity that can be corrected by surgery be apparent to the surgeon.

In some cases social and occupational failure, as well as emotional problems, are blamed on a cosmetic defect that is merely a scapegoat for deep, underlying psychological problems. Disturbances of this nature do not necessarily exclude cosmetic surgery, but as surgery alone is unlikely to solve the problem, the surgeon must proceed with caution. In most of these instances, as well as in other cases where the surgeon is unable to develop a comfortable understanding of the patient's motives, consultation with a psychiatrist or psychologist may be recommended before he accepts the patient for surgery (see chapter 3).

Perhaps the most important decision that the surgeon attempts to make during the interview is whether or not the candidate's assessment of his situation, and his motives and expectations from surgery are realistic. The patient must, above all, understand that facial cosmetic surgery is performed to produce improvement in appearance rather than perfection.

Preparation for
Cosmetic Facial Surgery

After the initial interview with the surgeon, the candidate

is either accepted for, or discouraged from, proceeding with cosmetic surgery. If the surgeon does not feel the operation is indicated, he will usually explain his reasons for this determination. Some patients are tentatively accepted for surgery, with the final decision made after consultation with other medical specialists or after additional interviews.

After he is accepted for cosmetic surgery, medical photographs of the patient are taken. These photographs are usually taken without makeup and are intended to provide a detailed record of the preoperative appearance of the patient. During a second preoperative visit, the surgeon carefully reviews these photographs with the patient, particularly emphasizing associated defects and facial asymmetries of which the patient may not be aware. Failure to point out such areas preoperatively may result in disappointment and dissatisfaction during the postoperative period when the patient is likely to carefully scrutinize his entire face.

For similar reasons, the location and extent of scars that may be produced by the operation are carefully discussed, and the process of wound healing and scar maturation are reviewed (see chapter 7).

Important details of the surgical procedure and postoperative care, including the surgeon's expectations of the patient during this period, are discussed. Possible complications are explained, and then an informed consent agreement giving permission for the surgeon to perform the operation is executed. Recent investigations of informed consent agreements have shown that patients remember only 20 to 30 percent of the information discussed during preoperative interviews. For this reason, some surgeons prefer to tape-record counselling sessions with patients. Literature detailing the material discussed with the patient may also be provided.

Fees for Cosmetic Facial Surgery

Fees for cosmetic facial surgery are generally paid in advance, and the surgeon or a member of his office staff discusses this matter with the patient before scheduling surgery. There are several reasons for requiring advance payment. Perhaps the most important of these is that advance payment insures that the patient has carefully considered the operation and is serious about having surgery. Such a patient will make careful arrangements to accommodate the procedure and is much less likely to suddenly cancel or request postponement of the operation for frivolous reasons several days before surgery. Cosmetic facial surgeons frequently have long waiting lists for operations and sudden cancellations make it extremely difficult for them to fill vacancies in their schedules on short notice. The surgical fee is refunded, of course, if the patient does change his mind at any time for any reason.

Additional Instructions
Given Before Surgery

The patient is instructed to avoid the use of aspirin or medications prescribed for other conditions that interfere with the clotting mechanism of the blood and thus may predispose to postoperative bleeding. Some surgeons prefer to avoid performing cosmetic surgery on women during the menstrual period as increased operative bleeding may occur at this time. The patient may also be instructed to wash his face or shampoo with a surgical detergent for several days before surgery to minimize the chance of infection.

Hospital or Office Surgery

If the operation is to be performed in a hospital, the patient is frequently admitted the evening before to undergo various laboratory procedures, X rays, EKG, etc., as indicated. An increasing number of cosmetic facial operations, however, are being performed in outpatient surgical facilities that the patient enters on the day of surgery and is discharged from, after a postoperative recovery period of several hours (see chapter 5). If surgery is scheduled in this manner, the patient is usually told to avoid solid food for six to eight hours before the operation to minimize the chance of nausea and vomiting.

Preoperative Medication

The patient is sedated one to two hours before surgery. Upon his arrival in the operating room, an intravenous infusion is started to allow supplemental medication to be administered as indicated. Electrodes for instruments that monitor cardiac activity and blood pressure during the operation are then connected.

Anesthesia for Cosmetic Facial Surgery

Most cosmetic facial operations are performed under local anesthesia. If this is the case, the anesthetic solution is infiltrated into the operative field with a small hypodermic needle. If the operation is to be performed under general anesthesia, an anesthesiologist will be present (see chapter 6).

Postoperative Care

After the surgical procedure is completed, the patient is returned to a special recovery area. If surgery was performed on an outpatient basis, the patient is driven home by a friend or relative after recovering from sedation. Postoperative instructions will depend on the type of surgery performed. They will be discussed later in conjunction with descriptions of each cosmetic surgical operation.

2

Concepts of Beauty

The shape of the face and the relationships between its features have been the objects of scrutiny since ancient times. In spite of the effort devoted to the study of beauty, no mathematical equation has been formulated for construction of a beautiful face. This is consistent with the belief that beauty exists in many forms and that many beautiful faces exhibit imperfections in one or more of their features.

Beauty seems to be an intuitive appreciation of balance, harmony and symmetry. We recognize beauty when we see it, but are unable to describe it in concrete or mathematical terms.

Even though "beauty is in the eyes of the beholder," the degree of agreement between people who recognize beauty is striking. Studies of preferences in feminine beauty that utilized both photographs and works of art have shown that judgment of beauty is remarkably constant in Western culture. Such uniformity of opinion is not surprising when one considers the universal appeal of certain movie stars, models, and beauty queens. No comparable studies of handsome males have been made, but the results would undoubtedly be similar.

As beauty cannot be defined mathematically, perhaps the best way to further explore this concept is to review the principles of facial balance, symmetry, harmony, and proportion originally devised by the ancient Greeks and Romans. These principles are still used by artists and sculptors as basic rules for construction of the face. Such an analysis is also important to facial surgeons because the extent to which certain facial features can or should be modified may depend on the relationship of the feature to the face as a whole. An understanding of facial proportions may also lead the surgeon to suggest modification of one or more features in addition to the one that the patient wants altered. He might, for instance, recommend increasing or decreasing the size of the chin in conjunction with cosmetic nasal surgery, or elevating the eyebrow in association with eyelid surgery. Proper hairstyling and use of cosmetics also depends on a fundamental appreciation of facial balance and symmetry.

Proportion in the Human Face

Proportion refers to the relative size or dimension of adjacent areas. The shape of the human face is somewhat oval. Variations include the square, round, or triangular face (fig. 1). The head is divided into two equal parts by a line drawn through the upper eyelids (fig. 2). These upper and lower segments of the ideal face are equally divided by a line drawn through the lowest part of the hairline and a line drawn through the junction of the nose and upper lip (fig. 2).

In the lower third of the face, the junction of the upper and lower lip lies at a point one-third of the distance between the base of the nose and chin. The edge of the ideal mouth touches lines drawn from the inner edge of each iris (fig. 3). The upper lip is somewhat thicker and more prominent than the lower lip. The junction of the upper lip's mucous membrane (red portion) with the skin in its central portion undulates in the shape of a flared "M," forming the Cupid's bow (fig. 4).

The width of each eye approximates the width of the nasal base and the distance between the inner edge of each eye is equal to the width of the eye (fig. 3). The outer edge of the beautiful eye is slightly higher than the inner edge, producing an upward slant. The eyebrow also slants upward, reaching

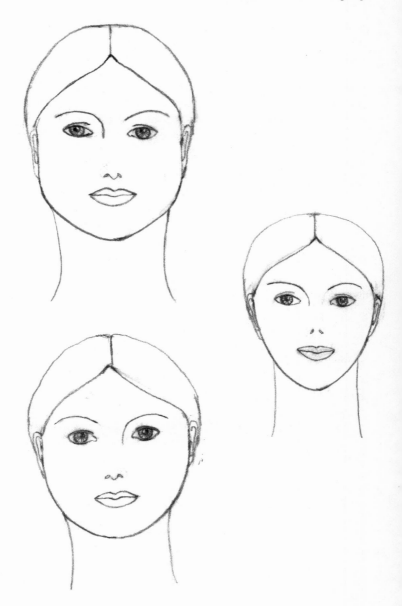

Fig. 1. Basic variations in facial configuration.

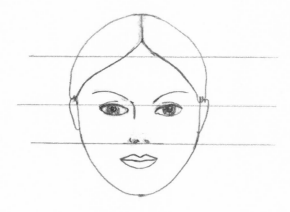

Fig. 2. Facial proportion.

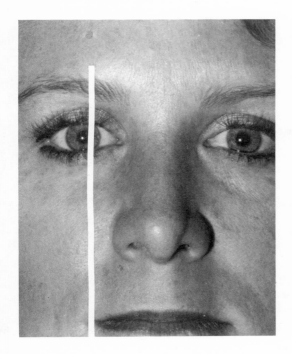

Fig. 3. The edges of the lips are on a tangent to lines drawn from the inner edge of each pupil. The width of the eye approximates the width of the base of the nose.

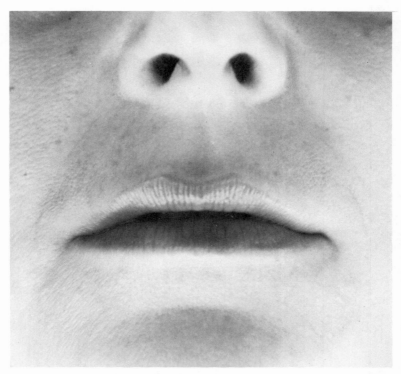

Fig. 4. "Cupid's bow:" the upper lip is more prominent than the lower.

its highest point at the outer edge of the iris, then descending somewhat.

The nose is the focal point of the middle third of the face, occupying its entire length. It is in the center of the face, and is widest at its base, approximately as wide as each eye. The base of the ideal nose is the shape of an equilateral triangle (fig. 5). The nostrils are just visible from the front and are oriented obliquely rather than horizontally or vertically (fig. 4).

The ears vary in size but are generally attached at a point just above the upper eyelid and parallel to the base of the nose (fig. 6). The upper half of the ear protrudes a greater distance from the head than the lower portion (fig. 2).

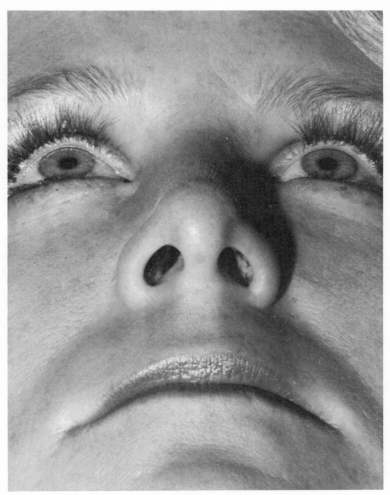

Fig. 5. The base of the nose forms an equilateral triangle.

How to Determine Facial Balance

Facial balance is determined by the relationships of various areas of the face (usually the upper, middle, and lower thirds) to each other. In the beautiful face, each third of the face contributes equally to the integral appearance. In such a

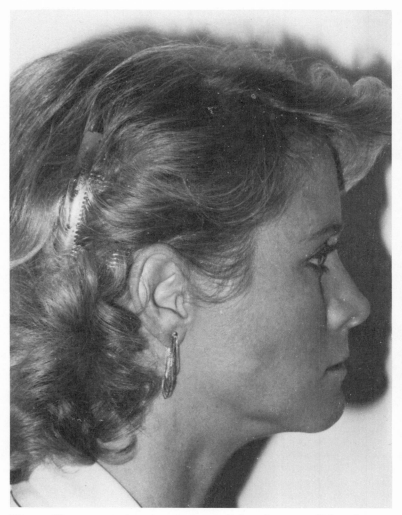

Fig. 6. The ear attaches at points parallel to the upper lid and nasal bone.

face each segment balances the other segments rather than draws attention to itself. One method of assessing facial balance is by constructing a "profile line" (fig. 6). The most prominent part of the upper and lower thirds of the face (i.e., the forehead and chin) should lie on a tangent to this line. The nose projects 30 to 36 degrees from the profile line. If the most prominent part of the upper and lower facial segments projects beyond or behind the profile line, facial balance is not ideal.

The Importance of Facial Harmony

Facial harmony implies an orderly and pleasing arrangement of the components of the face. In profile, the features of a beautiful face show regularity and gentle, graceful curves. Irregularities such as a nasal hump, excessive chin prominence, protruding lips, or a double chin distract from the harmonious relationship and draw attention away from the orderly and graceful arrangement of the rest of the face.

Symmetry in the Face

Symmetry implies a relationship in size, form, and arrangement between each half of the face. No human face is perfectly symmetrical, and mild asymmetry does not normally interfere with the perception of beauty. A greater degree of asymmetry, however, draws attention and thus detracts from the overall facial appearance.

The Anatomy of Beauty

Perhaps the most important anatomic component of the beautiful face is the structure of the facial bones. This skeletal framework is of vital importance in determining the shape of the forehead, nose, and chin, which to a large extent determine facial balance and harmony. Cosmetic surgery of the nose (chapter 14) and ears (chapter 17) and jaws (chapter 16) is largely directed toward modification of the skeletal structure of these features. Successful face-lift surgery (chapter 11) depends to a considerable extent on a favorable facial skeleton.

The muscles affecting facial expression may play a significant role in facial symmetry. These muscles are usually more active (or dominant) on one side of the face than on the other. Examples include the asymmetric smile and asymmetry of the eyes during various forms of facial expression.

The structure of the skin is also of considerable importance in the beautiful face. Redundant, sagging skin may obliterate the smooth, graceful curves of the facial profile.

The anatomy of beauty is closely related to the concepts of facial proportion, balance, harmony, and symmetry we have discussed. In the words of one prominent cosmetic surgeon, "beauty is often a matter of millimeters."

Is Beauty Really Important?

The old adage "beauty is only skin deep" suggests that the importance of physical attractiveness is often overestimated. Studies by social psychologists suggest that the physical appearance of a person is one of the most important components in the initial appeal or attraction he has for other people. After this initial impression, however, other factors tend to replace appearance in determining the type of relationship that ultimately develops. An individual's "self-image" is a major factor in determining his economic and psychosocial success in modern society, and perception of physical appearance is a major component of the self-image.

But even though physical attractiveness is certainly not the most important factor in interpersonal relationships, the value and importance of "looking one's best" has become increasingly apparent to many people. The increased emphasis on grooming aids, cosmetics, hairstyling, and fashion, as well as cosmetic surgery, attests to this trend.

3

Relationships Between Cosmetic Facial Surgery and Psychiatry

The profound psychological effect of facial abnormalities is well recognized. As such defects are difficult or impossible to conceal or camouflage, facial deformities exert a more significant influence on a person's self-image than do abnormalities on other areas of the body. Thus defects that seem to be within normal limits to a casual observer may disturb the self-image of an otherwise well-adjusted person to a degree that seems out of proportion to the magnitude of the deformity. Although it is generally assumed the extent of emotional imbalance attributed to a facial defect is in proportion to the extent of the abnormality, one study of patients undergoing cosmetic facial surgery showed no relationship between these factors. Contrary to popular opinion, no differences in emotional adjustment were found in this study between men and women accepted for cosmetic nasal surgery.

Regardless of the extent of a facial defect, poor adjustment or excessive concern over the defect may undermine a person's self-confidence and thus impair his performance and relationships with others. Such a person may feel that the defect is obvious enough to divert attention from his other qualities. The mannerisms and temporary withdrawal of adolescents and young adults after developing a prominent "pimple" or other embarrassing facial blemish provide a graphic illustration of this concept. When patients are properly selected, successful cosmetic surgery may significantly improve their self-image, outlook on life, and social adjustment.

Some people, however, tend to blame all of their failures on facial defects. Such behavior, of course, is usually unrealistic and cosmetic surgery is unlikely to resolve the deep emotional problems responsible for these feelings.

It is the task of the cosmetic surgeon to recognize this kind of patient and obtain further psychological evaluation before making a decision about surgery.

Historical Considerations

Since the inception of cosmetic surgery, its close relationship to psychiatry has been apparent. Controversy, however, has raged between these disciplines, concerning the advisibility of such surgery and its ultimate effect on the psyche. As recently as 1956, an article in a major surgical journal stated that "beauty surgery" for minor defects, including those that occur as a consequence of aging, was usually sought by people who were emotionally immature or maladjusted.

A corollary of this opinion was that the desire for cosmetic surgery was merely a superficial symptom of a deep underlying emotional disorder. Removal of such a surrogate symptom would only be followed by development of another symptom into which a patient could funnel his anxiety.

Consequently, medical opinion at this time held that cosmetic surgery should rarely be performed without psychiatric evaluation and clearance. As the field of cosmetic surgery expanded, this stance was gradually modified.

According to the new concept, patients requesting cosmetic surgery could be divided into two major groups. People with obvious major defects were thought to exhibit a low degree of emotional maladjustment and in general, were considered good candidates for surgery. People with "minimal" defects, on the other hand, were thought to have deeper underlying emotional disorders—the physical defect serving as a scapegoat for these problems. These people were advised to undergo psychological evaluation before cosmetic surgery.

As has been discussed, recent studies suggest that in many cases there is no relationship between the magnitude of a facial defect and the underlying emotional imbalance. This does not apply to people with deformities that are outside the normal range (see definition of cosmetic surgery, chapter 1).

In contemporary society, the desire to improve one's appearance is generally accepted as a normal characteristic. It is now apparent that appearance—particularly the facial appearance—is a major factor in a person's self-image.

As the attitudes of society toward cosmetic surgery changed, the psychiatric concept of the role of this type of surgical treatment in dealing with emotional problems underwent further modification. It is well recognized that several hours of surgery cannot eradicate all emotional conflicts that might otherwise require months or years of intensive psychotherapy. Nevertheless, it is now realized that appropriate use of cosmetic procedures can make a significant difference in the self-image and in other intangible factors that are intimately related to the self-image, such as self-confidence and outlook on life. The results of cosmetic facial surgery have supported this new concept. Studies have shown that a significant percentage of patients undergoing cosmetic facial surgery are satisfied with the results. For such patients, cosmetic facial surgery may provide a welcome charge of emotional energy and may bolster sagging self-esteem. Fortunately for the average candidate, scapegoating of symptoms has proven to be more of a theory than a practical concern.

Some patients, however, are displeased with the results of technically successful surgery and obtain no significant emotional benefits. Currently, emphasis is directed toward proper preoperative assessment and selection of candidates in order to avoid performing surgery on emotionally unstable people. The surgeon's task is to recognize such patients during preoperative interviews without subjecting each candidate to formal psychiatric evaluation.

The Preoperative Interview

During preoperative discussions with a prospective patient, the surgeon attempts to determine several basic things so he can evaluate which patients are likely to benefit from cosmetic surgery.

An important factor is the candidate's reason or motive for considering surgery. Contrary to popular belief, the surgeon does not expect an elaborate rationalization; he is seeking an honest and direct answer. People often seem reluctant to simply state that they want to improve their appearance, but in many cases this is entirely satisfactory to the surgeon.

In further analyzing the motivation for surgery, the surgeon attempts to determine its source. The motivation should come from the patient's inner feelings about his facial defect and should not stem entirely from a desire to please a husband, wife, friend, or relative. The desire for surgery, of course, should be discussed with those intimately related to the patient and should certainly be approved by them.

A desire to succeed in an occupation that involves dealing with the public is often a satisfactory motive, but such candidates must realize that in many cases deficiencies other than those for which they want surgery are often responsible for failure.

Another important factor in assessing motivation is the length of time that a patient has thought about correcting the facial defect. Ideally, a candidate will have considered surgery for a reasonable period of time before consulting a surgeon. People who request cosmetic surgery on the spur of the moment because of a sudden whim or emotional crisis—such as rejection by a boyfriend or a faltering marriage—are often poor candidates. Such people frequently adjust to these situations and then no longer feel a need for surgery.

A brief discussion of the candidate's current life situation is helpful in providing insight into motivational factors. It may also ease the tension of the interview, helping to establish the rapport between patient and surgeon that is necessary for a satisfactory culmination of the operative and postoperative period.

Another important factor in assessing the suitability of a person for facial cosmetic surgery is a determination of the patient's expectations. Again, the surgeon does not expect a complex rationalization. A frank, honest answer such as "I want to improve my appearance" is often satisfactory. The most important consideration is that the expectations be realistic. Does the prospective patient realize that although cosmetic facial surgery may improve his appearance, it will not solve all of his personal, social, or economic problems?

Does the patient realize the limitations of the operation itself? As has been noted, the surgeon is limited by the facial characteristics with which he must work, and he cannot remodel facial structures to the exact specifications of the patient. The candidate must realize that the goal of cosmetic facial surgery is improvement rather than perfection. This is particularly important in view of the recent glamorization of cosmetic surgery that has resulted in misconceptions and myths about this field.

A third factor that the surgeon attempts to evaluate is the general emotional makeup of the prospective patient. Some surgeons ask patients to complete a standard personality inventory form to assist in this evaluation while others rely on impressions formed during the interview. It is important for the surgeon to determine if the patient can successfully cope with the stresses of surgery and the postoperative healing period and if he can adjust to the possibility of a final result that falls short of his expectations. The surgeon also notes individual personality traits that may suggest that a more comprehensive psychological evaluation should be undertaken before surgery. Obvious examples of such personalities are the demanding or hostile individual, the overly secretive, or the hypochondriacal or obviously depressed person.

Although the specific questions and methods of interview used by cosmetic facial surgeons in patient interviews vary widely, the object of these preoperative interviews is to assess these factors.

Referral to a Psychiatrist
or Psychologist

The phenomenal success of cosmetic facial surgery supports the concept that many emotional problems related to facial defects may undergo significant resolution after successful surgery; yet there is no question that people with more serious psychological problems should be carefully evaluated before acceptance for surgery. As the surgeon is not equipped to conduct this evaluation, he often recommends referral to a psychiatrist or psychologist.

The patient who is requested to undergo such an evaluation should not feel offended. He should realize that the surgeon is making a conscientious effort to insure that cosmetic surgery can be performed with the best possible conditions for success—both physically and emotionally.

Frequently psychiatric evaluation is requested because the surgeon is unsure of the actual motivation for surgery. Or, he may feel that a patient's expectations of surgery are unrealistic and that a discussion of the situation with a psychiatrist or psychologist may help clarify or place the expectations in proper perspective.

In some cases it may be necessary to evaluate potentially unhealthy personality traits detected during the interview. Although such personality factors do not necessarily exclude a patient from undergoing cosmetic surgery, they may foster an emotional climate that prevents establishment of proper rapport between patient and surgeon. This lack of rapport may lead to misunderstandings that may compromise the surgical result. If the surgeon feels that an emotional rapport cannot be established with a particular surgical candidate, he will generally decline to accept the patient or will recommend consultation with a psychiatrist or another surgeon with whom he may develop a more favorable relationship.

Patients with facial defects that are so minor that the surgeon does not feel that correction is necessary may also present a problem. Such individuals often magnify minor or nonexistent defects out of proportion, blaming them for their failures in life. Several cosmetic surgeons have frequently been consulted about correction. Psychiatric evaluation is mandatory for these patients, but many patients refuse to accept this recommendation and continue to search for a surgeon who will satisfy their desire for surgery.

In most cases the psychiatric consultant is able to clarify motives and expectations, and the patient is accepted for cosmetic surgery. In other cases, a brief period of psychotherapy may be recommended prior to surgery in order to solve emotional conflicts. Then the operation can be undertaken with confidence.

Although the concepts governing the relationship between cosmetic surgery and psychiatry have undergone considerable change during the past decade, the fundamental association of facial deformities and the self-image will always necessitate a bond between these disciplines. Optimum results—both physical and emotional—can be expected only when this relationship is fully appreciated and exploited by surgeon, psychotherapist, and patient.

4

How to Choose a Cosmetic Facial Surgeon

The explosion of knowledge that has resulted in increasing degrees of specialization and subspecialization in modern medical practice has also had a major impact on the field of plastic surgery. The enormous proliferation of information and techniques relative to this field has made it difficult for the average surgeon to develop and maintain proficiency in all its aspects. Consequently, during the past twenty-five years physicians who specialize in surgical treatment of specific regions of the body have become proficient in the techniques of plastic surgery applicable to these particular regions.

Much of the momentum toward regionalization of plastic surgery has been generated by the specialty of *otolaryngology*— which deals with the diagnosis and treatment of diseases of the ear, nose, and throat, and other disorders of the head and neck. Many members of this surgical specialty have always concentrated on facial plastic and reconstructive surgery. However, because of major advances in preventing and treating diseases of the ear, nose, and throat, increasing numbers of physicians in this field have applied their abilities and expertise to the problems of plastic and reconstructive surgery of the head and neck.

There are other regional surgeons active in facial plastic surgery. The *ophthalmologist* (eye surgeon) may be proficient in plastic surgery of the eyelids and orbital region. *Dermatologists* may have special expertise in removing small facial tumors and blemishes as well as in other types of skin surgery such as hair transplantation. Oral surgeons are dental specialists who have made significant contributions to the field of orthognathic surgery. This field involves procedures designed to improve the form and function of the teeth and jaws, which are vitally important to the appearance of the lower third of the face (see chapter 16).

General plastic surgeons, certified in the specialty of plastic and reconstructive surgery, actively participate in cosmetic facial surgery. In addition to performing facial plastic surgery, these surgeons perform plastic surgery procedures on other areas of the body.

All the specialty groups involved in facial plastic and reconstructive surgery are represented by organized, official societies devoted to the exchange and dissemination of information and techniques as well as continuing education in the particular field. These organizations include the American Academy of Facial Plastic and Reconstructive Surgery, the American Academy of Otolaryngology and Head and Neck Surgery, the American Society of Plastic and Reconstructive Surgeons, the American Society for Aesthetic Plastic Surgery, the American Society of Oculoplastic and Reconstructive Surgery, the American Society for Dermatologic Surgery, and the American Academy of Oral and Maxillofacial Surgery.

Requirements for Certification

In order to better understand the qualifications of this diverse group of surgeons who may practice cosmetic facial surgery, a brief review of the requirements for certification in each specialty may be helpful.

OTOLARYNGOLOGY

Certification by the American Board of Otolaryngology requires four years of speciality training after graduation from medical school. During the first year, devoted to general surgery, the basic principles of all branches of surgery as well as pre- and postoperative management of patients undergoing major surgical procedures, are learned. Next, a three-year residency in diagnosis and medical and surgical treatment of disorders of the ear, nose, throat, head, and neck is completed. Such programs are required to provide the resident with training and experience in plastic and reconstructive surgery of the head and neck. After completing this four-year program, the resident must pass a written and oral examination administered by the American Board of Otolaryngology to become a board certified otolaryngologist. If he desires, he can complete another year of training in facial plastic and reconstructive surgery through a fellowship sponsored by the American Academy of Facial Plastic and Reconstructive Surgery.

OPHTHALMOLOGY

Certification by the American Board of Ophthalmology also requires four years of speciality training after graduation from medical school. The first year is spent as a resident in either general surgery or internal medicine and the next three years are devoted to study of diagnosis and management of eye diseases. During this period, the resident may gain experience in plastic surgery of the eye region and after completing his formal residency may elect to spend an additional year in a fellowship devoted to plastic and reconstructive surgery of the eye. Certification is achieved by passing a written and oral examination administered by the American Board of Ophthalmology.

DERMATOLOGY

Certification by the American Board of Dermatology requires one year of residency in internal medicine followed by three years of formal residency training in diagnosis and management of disorders of the skin. This includes experience in surgical excision of abnormalities of the facial skin. To be board certified, the physician must pass a written and oral examination.

GENERAL PLASTIC SURGERY

There are several routes to certification by the American

Board of Plastic Surgery. The most common path is three years of residency in general surgery followed by a two- or three-year training program in plastic and reconstructive surgery. Techniques and procedures for all regions of the body are taught. Certification is achieved by passing a written and oral examination administered by the American Board of Plastic Surgery.

Surgeons who are board certified in another surgical specialty are also eligible for admission to a plastic surgery residency. However, most of those who intend to limit their practices to facial or regional plastic surgery feel that additional training in techniques applicable to other areas of the body is unnecessary. If these surgeons desire further training in regional plastic surgery, one of the fellowship programs previously mentioned may be pursued.

ORAL SURGERY

After graduating from dental school, the prospective oral surgeon must complete a three-year residency program in this specialty. During this period, a substantial portion of his time may be devoted to diagnosis and treatment of deformities of the jaws, an area important to the appearance of the lower portion of the face. After completing this residency program, he must pass on oral and written examination for certification by the American Board of Oral Surgery.

Choosing a Facial Cosmetic Surgeon

The news media has focused considerable attention on unqualified and unscrupulous practitioners of cosmetic surgery. Perhaps as a consequence of these revelations, numerous articles on cosmetic surgery have appeared in newspapers and magazines and it has been widely covered on television and radio. Some of these discussions imply that only members of a certain specialty group are competent in this field—a contention that is misleading and groundless. As many surgeons in each of the specialties described possess the necessary credentials and expertise to perform cosmetic facial surgery, it is relatively unimportant whether the surgeon you choose is a regional plastic surgeon (otolaryngologist, ophthalmologist, dermatologist, oral surgeon) or a general plastic surgeon (plastic and reconstructive surgeon). By far the most important consideration is that the surgeon you choose has expertise in cosmetic facial surgery and, in particular, the surgical procedure in which you are interested. In keeping with the trend toward increasing specialization, some physicians limit their practice to one or more specific procedures; i.e., rhinoplasty, hair transplantation, or procedures for correction of facial aging.

The consumer should realize that cosmetic facial surgery constitutes only a small segment of the requirements for certification in each of the specialty groups with overlapping interests in this area. Thus, while board certification in one of these specialties may indicate that a surgeon has been exposed to the principles of cosmetic facial surgery during his residency training, board certification in itself is no guarantee of subsequent experience and proficiency in this field.

How then should the prospective candidate for cosmetic surgery choose a qualified surgeon? As with any major decision, one must exercise discretion and common sense in conducting his search. The following guidelines are suggested:

1. Although board certification in itself does not guarantee proficiency in cosmetic facial surgery, most reputable surgeons are certified by one of the specialty boards discussed. Your family physician or local medical society office may be able to provide names of cosmetic surgeons in your area.

2. Friends or acquaintances who have themselves undergone cosmetic surgery are an excellent source of information about doctors specializing in this area. Most cosmetic surgeons, in fact, find many new patients are referred by their previous patients. Most people who have had facial surgery are willing to discuss their experiences and will readily offer frank and candid opinions of their surgeons.

After you have selected a potential surgeon or surgeons, make an appointment for an evaluation of your particular problem. Prepare for your interview with the surgeon by making a list of specific questions about the nature and correction of your problem. Also, be prepared to ask about the qualifications and experience of the surgeon. Many patients are extremely passive during initial interviews and hesitate to question the surgeon about his qualifications and experience because they feel that such questions may irritate or insult the surgeon. Because of concern about unscrupulous practitioners, reputable surgeons encourage such discussions and are anxious to make patients aware of their qualifications. While no surgeon feels comfortable in an atmosphere of harsh interrogation, tactful questions about the following things are perfectly acceptable:

1. Specialty training and board certification or eligibility.
2. Membership in societies that promote continuing education in cosmetic surgery.
3. Experience in cosmetic facial surgery, especially in the particular procedure in which you are interested.
4. Privileges to perform the procedure in question in local hospitals. This is an important safeguard as many cosmetic operations are performed on outpatients in office operating rooms. While most reputable surgeons perform many of their facial procedures in office operating rooms, such surgery does not require approval by hospital surgical credentials committees. Evidence of privileges to perform the surgery in a hospital environment will insure that the credentials and experience of the surgeon have been evaluated by his peers and that he has demonstrated his competence to undertake such surgery.

All cosmetic surgeons maintain files of pre- and postoperative photographs of the procedures they perform. Many patients give their surgeons permission to show these photographs to surgery candidates so that they can better understand the benefits and limitations of various operations. Some surgeons, however, object to showing such photographs when the identity of the patient is revealed.

Regardless of the availability of pre- and postoperative photographs, you may want to speak with some of the surgeon's previous patients. Many surgeons maintain a list of people who are willing to discuss their experiences with prospective patients.

The search for cosmetic surgeons should not end with locating a qualified physician. It is important that you feel comfortable and at ease with him. As the preoperative preparation and postoperative care of the patient undergoing cosmetic facial surgery involves considerable personal interaction between patient and surgeon, and the personalities of both individuals can vary, you should be sure that you can establish an emotional rapport with your surgeon. Lack of such rapport is often the source of considerable personal anguish, misunderstanding, and even hostility—if the lines of communication are strained.

It is fortunate that the great demand for cosmetic facial surgery in modern society has stimulated the interest of the surgical specialists in various disciplines. The input and exchange of new ideas and techniques by these doctors will benefit the patient by encouraging advancement in this field.

5

Outpatient and Hospital Surgery

An increasing number of cosmetic facial surgeons are performing many of their operations in outpatient surgical facilities. This may seem somewhat unusual to the prospective patient as most people associate surgery with hospitalization. Dental surgeons, however, have performed operations on an outpatient basis for years, using both local and general anesthetics. Their experience has demonstrated the safety and efficiency of outpatient surgery and has been a factor in the trend toward the use of outpatient facilities for many nonemergency operations.

A study by the Government Accounting Office suggests that as many as 40 percent of surgical procedures now performed in hospital operating rooms can be done safely in outpatient facilities. When the patients are properly selected, cosmetic facial operations are ideal procedures for outpatient surgery as they are usually performed under local anesthesia, are relatively short in duration, and involve only the skin and subcutaneous tissues.

But why would a surgeon suggest performing an operation in an outpatient facility if hospital space is available? Perhaps the major advantage of outpatient surgery is its lower cost in the face of the rapidly ascending spiral of hospitalization and operating room fees. The cost of hospitalization for cosmetic surgery may approach that of the operation itself. As cosmetic facial surgery is rarely covered by health care insurance (although expenses are tax deductible), the patient usually bears the entire expense. Consequently, surgery performed on an outpatient basis saves him considerable money.

Outpatient surgery offers other advantages. Many people do not like hospitalization, especially when they are not sick. They are often less anxious about undergoing surgery in an outpatient facility and convalescing at home. For many, the convenience and privacy of outpatient surgery is appealing.

Outpatient surgery is advantageous for the surgeon too. It saves him the time and expense of commuting between office and hospital and relieves him of much of the paperwork of hospitalization.

Requirements for an Outpatient Surgery Facility

Certain basic requirements must be met for safe performance of outpatient surgery. The operating area must be equipped with instruments to monitor the patient's vital functions. Equipment and medications should be readily available to treat any emergency condition that may arise.

Not all patients undergoing cosmetic facial surgery are candidates for outpatient surgery. Most surgeons agree that those with a significant medical condition are more safely treated in a hospital operating room. In this environment, various medical specialists are available to assist in the treatment of any emergency situation. Nurses are present to watch for problems that may develop in the early postoperative period.

The safety of outpatient surgery has been documented by the experiences of both dental surgeons and cosmetic surgeons. Complication rates following outpatient cosmetic surgery are as low as those of operations performed in the hospital. With proper patient selection and use of local anesthesia, problems other than those related to anesthetic reactions are most unusual.

Two basic types of outpatient surgical facilities are widely used. Many hospitals and private health care corporations have constructed areas especially designed for outpatient surgery and are equipped to use either general or local anesthesia. Some surgeons have arranged to use hospital emergency room operating areas for outpatient surgery. The second type of outpatient facility is the office operating room. Both types meet the safety requirements discussed and are equipped with recovery areas where patients are observed for several hours after the operation. As considerable expense is involved in establishing and maintaining an office operating room, a small fee is usually charged for using it. This charge, however, is usually less than the fees for using other types of outpatient surgical areas.

The Outpatient Surgical Procedure

The patient who is to have outpatient cosmetic facial surgery arrives at the surgical unit or office on the day his operation is scheduled. Frequently the surgeon has provided a sedative for him to take at home several hours before surgery. An intravenous infusion is started, through which additional sedation is administered, and equipment to monitor the pulse and heart rhythm is connected. The local anesthetic is then administered and the operation performed.

After the surgery, the patient is transferred to the recovery area where she or he is observed by the nurse and surgeon for several hours. A companion then drives the patient home. The surgeon usually phones the patient on the evening of surgery and on the first postoperative day to insure that convalescence is satisfactory. The patient then returns to the surgeon's office for postoperative care.

As has been noted, the rate of complications following cosmetic facial surgery performed on an outpatient basis is almost identical to that after hospital surgery. Surveys of patients who have had outpatient cosmetic surgery show that most have been pleased with their experiences and would recommend outpatient surgery to others.

6

Anesthesia for Cosmetic Facial Surgery

Adequate anesthesia—defined as loss of sensation in a part of the body or in the entire body as the result of the administration of a drug (the anesthetic)—is an obvious prerequisite for performance of surgery in a manner satisfactory to both doctor and patient. Much of the success of contemporary surgery is related to advances in the safety and effectiveness of anesthesia, and the development of safe and reliable anesthetic techniques has, to a large extent, facilitated the acceptance and more frequent use of cosmetic facial surgery.

The goals of anesthesia are relief of pain and protection of the vital functions of the body during surgery.

Types of Anesthesia

Anesthesia can be divided into two major classes—general and local. Local anesthesia, in which loss of sensation is confined to the part of the body on which surgery is to be performed, is obtained by infiltration or topical application of an anesthetic agent. General anesthesia, which involves the entire body, is induced by inhalation or intravenous injection of an anesthetic. General anesthesia results in unconsciousness and depression of vital cardiovascular (heart) and pulmonary (lung) functions. Thus it necessitates careful monitoring and support of these functions. This usually means a tube must be placed through the nose or mouth into the trachea (an *endotracheal* tube) in order to allow the anesthetist to control the patient's breathing.

Although some surgeons perform cosmetic facial surgery under general anesthesia, most of these procedures are performed under local anesthesia. The most important reason for this is that cosmetic facial surgery is elective; i.e., neither life nor an important organ of the body is in jeopardy and although the risk of general anesthesia is low, local anesthesia is safer.

Local Anesthesia

Local anesthetics block perception of pain by interfering with the activity of nerve fibers, which conduct pain impulses to the brain. Today these agents must be injected into the tissues with a small hypodermic needle, but methods of administering local anesthetics through the intact skin by means of electrical currents (*iontophoresis*) are being developed and these techniques may be available to surgeons in the future.

Anesthetic agents can, however, be applied topically to the mucous membranes of the nose to help obtain anesthesia for nasal surgery.

Local anesthetics are identified by the suffix -caine and commonly used agents include lidocaine, carbocaine, and tetracaine. Cocaine is often used for topical anesthesia of the nasal mucous membranes, but is never injected into tissues. An advantage of cocaine is its ability to induce constriction of blood vessels and significantly decrease operative bleeding.

Adrenalin is usually added to local anesthetics (except in the case of cocaine) used in cosmetic facial surgery for two reasons. It causes constriction of blood vessels, decreasing operative bleeding. It also prolongs the duration of the anesthesia, increasing the time available for surgery to one-and-one-half to two hours.

Reactions to Local Anesthesia

Although local anesthesia is extremely safe, it is not entirely without risk. Most people have probably heard stories of "reactions" to local anesthetics from their friends or relatives. The majority of these "reactions" are the result of *syncopal* episodes (fainting spells) secondary to apprehension associated with injections in sensitive areas. Adrenalin in the anesthesic causes rapid and forceful beating of the heart, which may precipitate apprehension interpreted as a "reaction."

True adverse reactions to local anesthetics are most frequently due to an overdose. Safe doses for all anesthetic agents are well established and the surgeon will stay within this safe range. Occasionally, however, a patient is abnormally sensitive to these drugs, and develops a true toxic reaction after administration of a dose within the recommended range. Such a toxic reaction is usually manifested by restlessness and excitability, which may turn into convulsions. In the case of a severe overdosage, depression of the cardiovascular system and unconsciousness may occur. If promptly recognized, these reactions are easily treated and subside without harm to the patient. Equipment and medicines used to treat anesthetic reactions are available in all operating rooms where cosmetic facial surgery is performed (see chapter 5). In addition, sophisticated devices to monitor the patient's vital functions are used during all operations performed under local anesthesia.

In extremely rare cases, a patient may be allergic to the agent. Although true allergy to older local anesthetic agents (most commonly procaine) did occur, such reactions to the newer anesthetics, which are of a different chemical structure, are unusual. Most experienced surgeons and anesthesiologists indicate that they have never had a patient who experienced a true "allergic reaction" to these anesthetics. On occasion, a person may be allergic to a chemical preservative in the solution. If a patient states that he is "allergic" to the anesthetic that the surgeon wants to use, skin testing procedures may be used to determine the presence or absence of an allergic state. In most such cases, however, another agent is used.

A patient who experiences adverse reactions to local anesthetics should ask his surgeon to clarify the nature of this reaction in his medical records so that he does not erroneously think himself "allergic" to the drug, and unnecessarily deprive himself of a safe and useful agent.

Adjuncts to Local Anesthesia

It is natural for a patient to be apprehensive about any surgical procedure as well as about the administration of a local anesthetic. The emotional rapport that the surgeon establishes with his patient during the preoperative period can do much to allay such anxiety. Careful explanation of each step during administration of the anesthetic as well as frequent reassurance that all is going well are also extremely helpful in reducing apprehension.

Before he arrives in the operating room, the patient is given various sedatives and pain-relieving agents. If necessary, additional amounts of these medications are given with an intravenous line established in the operating room. This intravenous line also provides a route for rapid administration of drugs if there is an adverse reaction to the anesthetic or other medications.

In most cases, the patient undergoing cosmetic facial surgery under local anesthesia with sedation is pleasantly surprised by the ease of the situation. Often he dozes in a twilight zone and has little recollection of the procedure.

General Anesthesia

General anesthesia is a state of unconsciousness in which pain impulses are not perceived. As depression of cardiovascular and pulmonary function also occurs with general anesthesia, these functions must be carefully monitored and supported during the operation. In most cases, the anesthetist must breathe for the patient through a tube placed through the mouth or nose into the trachea (an endotracheal tube).

General anesthetics consist of gases which are administered via a mask or tube, and medications that are given intravenously. In most cases, anesthesia is initially induced by intravenous medications, and after placement of an endotracheal tube, the anesthetist continues with gaseous agents. These general anesthetics are frequently supplemented by various muscle-relaxing drugs.

Although many patients think that they would prefer general anesthesia for cosmetic facial surgery, most surgeons prefer local anesthesia. Some surgeons will perform these operations under general anesthesia, but others refuse to operate unless the patient agrees to a local anesthetic. The potential disadvantages of general anesthesia for cosmetic facial surgery are numerous. The elective nature of these operations is obvious and has been discussed previously.

A major consideration is bleeding. Most general anesthetics dilate blood vessels and thus increase bleeding in the operative field. Although such bleeding would not ordinarily cause an excessive operative blood loss, it may interfere with the surgeon's performance and increase operative time. The possibility of postoperative bleeding may also be increased. Although adrenalin can be infiltrated into the operative site to counteract this vascular dilation, it is usually not as effective as when used with local anesthetics. Also, some general anesthetics sensitize the heart to adrenalin, and use of this agent in such circumstances may produce serious irregularities in the heartbeat.

Operative bleeding during general anesthesia can be minimized by the technique of *hypotensive anesthesia* in which the blood pressure is maintained at lower than normal levels. Although this technique is safe when used by a skilled anesthesiologist, the risk is probably somewhat higher than in routine forms of general anesthesia.

Another disadvantage of general anesthesia in cosmetic facial surgery is the inability of the patient to cooperate with the surgeon during the operation. During most operations the patient can help the surgeon by moving into positions that facilitate surgery. Moving the unconscious patient is more difficult and entails a small risk of dislodging the endotracheal tube or monitoring devices.

The endotracheal tube may interfere with the surgeon's perception of the relationship of the various facial structures, which is important to proper execution of the procedure, particularly in cosmetic nasal surgery.

Some surgeons feel that the positive pressure required to breathe for the patient through the endotracheal tube may increase the venous pressure at the operative site, predisposing to operative and postoperative bleeding. Such bleeding may lead to troublesome accumulation of blood beneath the skin in the postoperative period. Similarly, coughing, retching, and even vomiting is not uncommon when emerging from general anesthesia. Such involuntary reflexes also increase venous pressure and the probability of postoperative bleeding.

In spite of these objections, cosmetic facial surgery can be satisfactorily performed under general anesthesia if for some reason local anesthesia cannot be tolerated. The patient is counselled about these potential problems and prepared to accept the risks of their occurrence.

Although the goals of anesthesia for cosmetic facial surgery—relief of pain and safety—are best satisfied by a local anesthetic with supplemental sedation, it would be unfair to state that general anesthesia, in spite of its disadvantages, does not play a viable role in cosmetic facial surgery. After a careful discussion of the advantages and disadvantages of each method, most patients elect local anesthesia. Those who insist on a general anesthetic, however, can undergo surgery with confidence that the procedure will be just as successful.

7

Wound Healing and Scar Formation

Contrary to popular opinion, the cosmetic surgeon cannot make an incision in the facial skin without producing a scar. Every wound that penetrates the dermal layer of the skin, regardless of the way it is produced, results in a scar. While scars that form after accidents and injuries are frequently unsightly, incisions used in cosmetic facial surgery are carefully planned so that the resulting scar is minimized. This chapter will focus on the process of wound healing and maturation, as well as on the techniques used by the cosmetic facial surgeon to minimize and hide scars.

The Process of Wound Healing

All wounds heal the same way regardless of their extent and location. Wound healing is initiated by inflammation. Small blood vessels in the injured area dilate, transporting white blood cells, antibodies, and other chemical substances that combat infection. The blood-clotting mechanism is activated and a small clot forms over the wound, protecting it from further contamination. Cells called *macrophages* remove contaminants from the wound. In surgical incisions contamination is slight, and thus the inflammatory reaction is minimized. In many traumatic wounds, however, this phase is intense and prolonged because of excessive contamination and infection. Proper emergency treatment of such wounds hastens healing and minimizes the resulting scar.

After contamination and infection are controlled, cells called *fibroblasts* appear in the injured area and produce fibers of *collagen*, a protein material that is the basic structural building block of the body. Collagen production begins on the fourth or fifth day after injury and continues for two to four weeks depending on the extent of the wound. These collagen fibers aggregate into bundles that fill the defect between the injured surfaces and provide tensile strength for the wound.

During the period of collagen production, the surface of the wound heals by migration of *epithelial* cells from the skin surface (*epidermis*) across the defect, a process called *epithelialization*. In the case of surgical incisions, this surface healing is completed in one or two days, but it takes longer in larger wounds.

The scar produced by the initial processes is a bulky, soft, fragile, and loosely organized structure with a red appearance. It is often elevated from the skin's surface. The period during which the scar changes to assume its final appearance is called the phase of maturation. During this period, collagen fibers become arranged into patterns that increase the tensile strength of the wound. This fiber orientation undergoes continuous change during maturation as it adapts to the stresses placed on the wound by surrounding tissue.

The bulk of the scar gradually decreases during this period, and as the small blood vessels that cause the red color of the immature scar disappear, the scar becomes whitish. The scar also exhibits a tendency to widen during maturation as a result of continuous stress placed on the wound by the surrounding tissues.

Scar maturation shows considerable individual variation and may take six months to two years. This process is usually more intense and prolonged in younger people. The length and intensity of scar maturation also varies in different areas and is related to the size of the original wound and the stresses placed on it. The end result of maturation is the dense, firm, white scar with which most people are familiar.

Factors That Retard Wound Healing

As is the case with any biologic or mechanical process, wound healing can be adversely affected by a number of factors. Poor nutrition compromises healing, as does deficiency of vitamin C, which plays a vital role in collagen production.

Diabetes is associated with impaired wound healing. Although this is more marked during the late stages of poorly controlled diabetes, in which small blood vessels become deficient, poorly understood metabolic abnormalities may compromise healing in young diabetics. People with advanced disease of the liver or kidney may also suffer impairment of wound healing.

Areas of the body that have been exposed to radiation heal poorly as a result of radiation-induced damage to small blood vessels.

Cortisone and cortisonelike medications also impair healing. They are frequently used in treatment of *hypertrophic scars* and *keloids*. People with overactivity of the glands that produce cortisone (Cushing's disease) are poor healers.

In spite of the considerable amount of time and effort devoted to research in this area, no factor that enhances or accelerates wound healing has been found. There is no evidence to support the contention that vitamin E improves healing.

Hypertrophic Scars and Keloids

An occasional wound heals with excessive production of collagen, forming a large, red, elevated scar called a hypertrophic scar (fig. 1). The exact reasons for this exuberant reaction are unknown, but it is recognized that hypertrophic scars are more common in dark-skinned people and occur more frequently on certain areas of the body, particularly the chest and upper back. Hypertrophic scarring is also more likely to occur when wounds are closed under excessive tension.

Continued proliferation of collagen in a scar results in formation of a keloid (fig. 2). The distinguishing feature of the

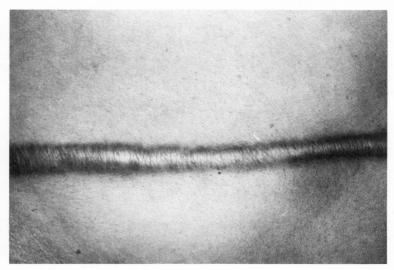

Fig. 1. A hypertrophic scar.

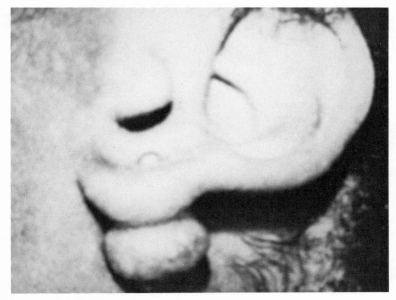

Fig. 2. A keloid.

keloid is its invasion of surrounding normal tissue. These scars occur most frequently in dark-skinned people and cause itching and sharp, intermittent pain, secondary to pressure on nerve endings. A common place for facial keloids is the *lobule* of the ear (fig. 2).

Factors That Determine the Magnitude of a Scar

Many factors are important in determining the extent of a cutaneous scar. Of considerable significance is the nature of the wounding agent. The surgical wound made with a clean, sharp scalpel causes less tissue injury than a laceration caused by a jagged piece of glass; thus, all other factors being equal, it produces a less noticeable scar. Contamination that occurs in a traumatic wound also invites a more vigorous and prolonged inflammatory response and predisposes to healing with a more significant scar. Surgical cleansing and closure of such a wound, of course, will result in a scar that is less conspicuous than one produced by spontaneous healing of the defect.

The area of incision is another important determinant in scarring. Wounds on the face characteristically heal with a finer scar than do wounds on the trunk or extremities.

The quality of skin in the injured area also plays an important role. Scars in areas covered with thick, oily skin—such as the nose—are more noticeable than those in areas of thin skin—such as the eyelids.

The orientation of the wound with respect to the natural lines of skin tension (fig. 3) is of extreme importance in determining the magnitude of scarring. Wounds that are parallel to these tension lines produce scars that are less perceptible than those resulting from wounds that cross these lines.

The degree of tension or tightness with which a wound is closed is important in the magnitude of the resulting scar. The surgical wound, the edges of which fall together with little tension, produces a less conspicuous scar than the traumatic wound associated with loss of a portion of skin that requires the surgeon to pull the edges together tightly to

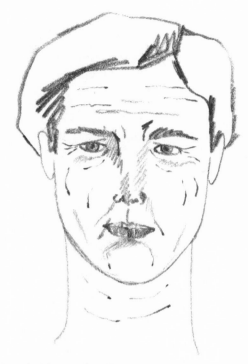

Fig. 3. Relaxed skin-tension lines.

obtain closure. Wounds occurring in areas of activity, such as the skin over the joints, are subject to constant tension from joint motion; thus they heal with larger scars than wounds in less active areas. As noted above, tension and stress are major factors contributing to hypertrophic scarring and keloid formation.

Age is also important. Scars tend to be more conspicuous in younger people. This is partly explained by the fact that skin becomes progressively more lax with increasing age, resulting in reduced tension on the healing wound.

Surgical technique, obviously, is an important factor in scar production. The carefully planned and executed surgical incision should heal with a less conspicuous scar than a poorly planned incision or traumatic laceration.

The cosmetic facial surgeon uses well-established techniques to minimize and camouflage scars from incisions he makes in the skin of the face. As noted previously, no surgeon can incise the skin without creating a scar. The concept that the plastic or cosmetic surgeon can operate without producing scars is a myth.

In planning incisions on the face, the cosmetic surgeon places these incisions in areas where the scars will be least conspicuous. In cosmetic nasal surgery, incisions are placed inside the nose, where they are not visible. External incisions are placed at the junctions of facial landmarks where small scars will be naturally camouflaged. Such junctions include the ear–face junction used for the face-lift operation and the eye–cheek junction sometimes used for excision of large lower eyelid "bags." Other external incisions are placed in the hairline or at the junction of the hairline and facial skin so that they can be covered by styling the hair. Facial incisions may also be hidden by placing them in the natural facial creases described in chapter 9.

In addition to carefully planning and placing incisions, the cosmetic facial surgeon uses certain techniques to enhance formation of a fine, narrow scar. Gentle handling of tissue is important in order to prevent needless injury that would make inflammation worse. Fine surgical instruments facilitate gentle handling of tissue. Bleeding is carefully and completely controlled to minimize the risk of postoperative hemorrhage, which is detrimental to healing. The wound edges are closed with fine suture material that minimizes the extent of foreign material in the wound. The edges are approximated without tension that would tend to strangulate the healing wound, predisposing to increased scarring.

After suture removal, many surgeons recommend supporting the healing wound with skin tapes that retard the widening of the scar that tends to occur before the wound develops enough tensile strength.

Although these techniques usually result in a narrow scar that is satisfactory to both patient and surgeon, complications of the healing process, many of which are beyond the control of the surgeon, can compromise the final result.

Revision of Scars

Although revision of facial scars is not within the sphere of cosmetic surgery according to the definition in chapter 1, it is an important part of the practice of many cosmetic facial surgeons and will be briefly discussed.

Scars can never be completely eliminated, and so the goal of scar revision is improvement rather than eradication. This must be understood and accepted by the patient, or scar revision results will not be satisfactory.

Of paramount importance in determining the advisability of scar revision is the age of the scar. Ideally the scar should have undergone complete maturation, which takes from six months to two years. Surgeons are often pressured to revise scars before this, but in most cases this is inadvisable as the appearance of the scar will improve with maturation. Also, revision is usually more successful after maturation, as less tissue is removed and the wound can be closed under less tension.

The age of the patient is also important, as it is related to scar maturation and skin tension as discussed.

The surgeon is also interested in the manner in which the scar was caused. Revision will be more satisfactory if the initial scar was produced in a traumatic, contaminated wound rather than in a clean surgical wound. The location of the scar is also important in assessing benefit from revision. Scars in thick, oily skin are easier to minimize than those in thin, dry skin.

The orientation of the scar with respect to the natural skin creases is important in predicting the extent of improvement following revision. Scars that are parallel to these creases are more easily treated than those that cross these lines.

The width and length of the scar are also important, as are such factors as elevation or depression in relation to the surrounding skin.

Psychological considerations are also important in assessing the candidate for scar revision. Scars are often reminders of significant episodes that have occurred earlier in the patient's life. They may be associated with feelings of anger, hostility, or shame. Parents of young children with facial

.

scars may harbor feelings of guilt about these deformities. The surgeon encourages the patient to express these feelings during preoperative interviews. If the surgeon feels that the patient has not satisfactorily resolved his emotional conflicts about the disfigurement, or that his expectations are not realistic, he may recommend psychiatric evaluation before surgery (see chapter 3).

The candidate for scar revision must also understand that several procedures may be required.

Techniques of Revision

The surgical technique selected to revise a scar depends on the location, length, width, and orientation of the scar. Short scars that are parallel to natural skin creases are frequently satisfactorily corrected by simple excision and reapproximation of the edges.

Longer scars and those crossing natural skin creases require more sophisticated methods. Long scars are easily followed by the eye, and the basic principle underlying revision of such scars is breaking this predictable pattern by changing the direction of the scar at frequent intervals along its length. Two methods frequently employed include the W-plasty (fig. 4) and the geometric line closure (fig. 5). While at first glance these methods seem radical, experience has shown that the resulting irregular scar is much less perceptible than the original regular one as it is less predictible to the eye.

Ancillary Measures in Scar Revision

Many surgeons recommend supporting the healing wound with skin tapes after suture removal in order to prevent widening of the scar. The maximum benefit is obtained by using these tapes for six weeks. During this period the wound acquires enough tensile strength to resist the surrounding stresses responsible for widening.

Dermabrasion (see chapter 20) is often helpful in smoothing surface irregularities between the scar and the surrounding skin. This procedure may be performed six to

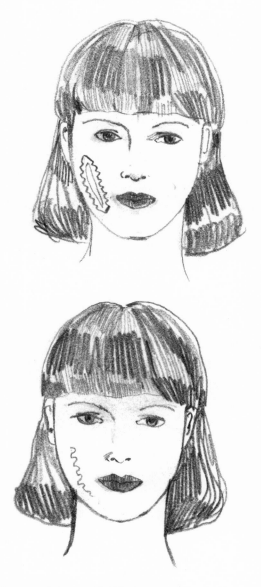

Fig. 4. Scar revisions with W-*plasty.*

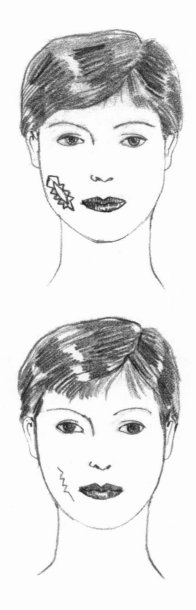

Fig. 5. Scar revision with geometric line closure.

twenty-four months after surgical revision of the scar, depending on its rate of maturation. Elimination of these small surface irregularities may make the scar less visible. In some cases surface irregularities can be improved by shaving high points with a surgical scalpel instead of using dermabrasion.

Judicious application of cosmetics is frequently of considerable benefit in camouflaging surgically revised scars. It is particularly useful during the early stages of healing and maturation when the wound tends to be elevated and red.

8

Facial Blemishes

Although removal of facial blemishes is not strictly within the realm of cosmetic surgery according to the definition discussed in chapter 1, many people who have them consult cosmetic facial surgeons for advice and treatment. Localized facial skin disorders can generally be classified as benign or malignant (cancerous). Although most facial blemishes are benign, many people consult a physician because they fear a malignancy. Skin cancer, however, except for the rare malignant *melanoma*, rarely occurs in young people or in older people who have not been exposed to the sun for many years (see chapter 10).

As the treatment of skin malignancies is not within the scope of cosmetic surgery, it will not be discussed in this book.

Methods of Treating Facial Blemishes
There are several satisfactory methods for dealing with facial blemishes. The method of treatment is determined by the type, size, and location of the growth, the wishes of the patient, and the training and experience of the physician consulted.

SURGICAL EXCISION

Surgical excision is perhaps the most frequently recommended method of treatment for facial blemishes and it is performed under local anesthesia in the surgeon's office. As a scar will result, the cosmetic surgeon carefully plans the procedure so that the scar will be oriented in the direction of the natural facial lines described in chapter 7. The usual orientation and shape of these incisions is diagrammed in figure 1.

The area of excision is usually planned so that it is elliptical in shape as a skin wound of this configuration is easily closed in a straight line.

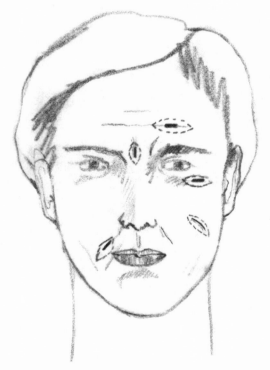

Fig. 1. Placement of incisions in natural skin creases helps hide scar.

Fundamental principles of plastic surgery are applied in an attempt to minimize the surgical scar. Small, sharp instruments are used and tissues are handled gently. Bleeding is carefully controlled before closing the wound. The surgeon separates the skin and subcutaneous fat from the underlying tissue (a technique called undermining) for a distance roughly equal to the width of the surgical defect. This is done to reduce tension on the skin edges that would encourage widening of the scar during the process of maturation (see chapter 7). The wound is then meticulously closed with fine sutures. Many surgeons place permanent, nonabsorbable sutures beneath the epidermal layer to provide tensile strength to combat the tendency of the scar to widen during maturation. As such sutures may later become infected and extrude from the wound, some surgeons prefer to use sutures that will be absorbed by the body.

An antibiotic ointment is then placed over the incision. This ointment tends to keep the surface of the wound moist and to prevent crusting of blood and other fluid that may leak from the incision during the first days of healing. The ointment, which the patient applies several times a day, also forms a film that protects the wound from contamination and combats bacteria that are on the skin surface, helping to prevent infection. Some surgeons prefer to place a small bandage or dressing over the wound instead of using ointment.

In most cases, the stitches in the wound surface are removed on the third to fifth postoperative day. At this time, the surgeon frequently applies skin tapes to support the wound during the early phase of healing when the tendency to widen is strongest.

As previously discussed, the scar tends to appear red during the first few months. As maturation proceeds, however, this color gradually fades and ultimately a fine, white scar is produced. (A detailed description of wound healing is presented in chapter 7.)

The principle advantage of removing facial blemishes by surgical excision is virtually complete eradication. A second advantage is that the area that is removed can be sent to a pathology laboratory for microscopic examination. Although most facial blemishes are accurately diagnosed by the physician, others, particularly *nevi* (moles) and abnormal skin growths in older people, must be examined by a pathologist to completely exclude the presence of a malignancy.

ALTERNATE METHODS

Many superficial skin disorders can be removed by other methods that, in many cases, are more rapid and less inconvenient to the patient and that produce little or no visible scarring. Often, a small portion of the abnormal area is removed and sent for microscopic examination before complete removal to provide an accurate diagnosis. If a malignancy is suspected or proven by this biopsy, the following techniques are usually abandoned in favor of surgical excision.

Many superficial blemishes can be shaved from the skin surface with a sharp blade—a procedure called shave excision. As only a portion of the skin under the abnormality is removed, healing generally occurs without formation of a visible scar. This procedure also allows the growth to be submitted for microscopic examination and thus a preoperative biopsy is not necessary.

A circular skin punch is also often used to remove small facial blemishes (fig. 2). This procedure is of particular

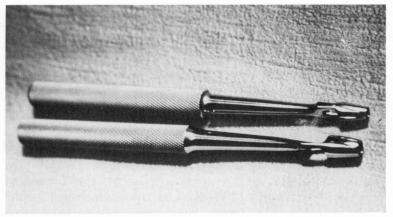

Fig. 2. Skin punch.

value in excising small *nevi* or moles. A punch just large
enough to fit around the mole is placed over the area and the
sharp edges of the punch remove the area, leaving a small
circular defect that can be closed with a suture or left to heal
spontaneously. Only a relatively inconspicuous, slightly pitted
scar is left. This method also provides a specimen for microscopic examination.

Sharp instruments called curettes are also used to remove
some skin abnormalities. Physicians skilled in this method
are able to distinguish abnormal tissue by feel and thus are
able to avoid significant removal of surrounding tissue. The
defect is allowed to heal spontaneously and produces a scar
similar to that caused by excision with a skin punch.

Some small facial blemishes are effectively eradicated by
electrical current, a process called *electrodesiccation* or *ful-
guration*. Unless the physician is certain of the nature of the
blemish, a surgical biopsy must be done before using this
method, as desiccation completely destroys the growth. Electrodesiccation is also frequently used in conjunction with
shave and punch excision to insure destruction of the base of
the lesion and to control bleeding. Some superficial skin lesions can be removed using dermabrasion (see chapter 20).

Skin blemishes caused by exposure to the sun over long
periods of time are frequently removed by a process called
chemosurgery. A chemical, most commonly the substance 5-
fluorouracil (5-FU), is applied to the area for a period of time.
This agent produces an intense skin redness, but is very
effective in removing these areas, which in many cases are
precancerous. Chemosurgery is occasionally performed with
weak acid solutions or phenol.

Superficial skin lesions are often treated with *cryosurgery*.
In this technique an application of extreme cold, usually in
the form of liquid nitrogen, is used for eradication.

Blemishes located just below the skin are sometimes
treated with surgical tatooing. In this process, flesh colored
pigments are placed into the skin in an attempt to camouflage the discoloration produced by the blemish (fig 3). Recently, surgeons have reported good results from using small
laser beams to eradicate some of these areas of discoloration.

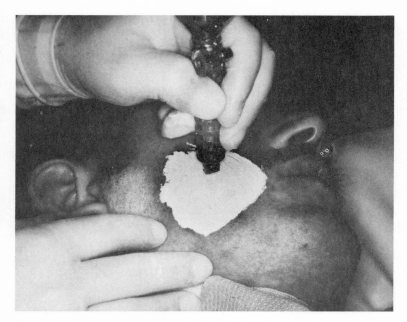

Fig. 3. Surgical tatooing.

Common Superficial Skin Blemishes

A multitude of skin disorders can cause facial blemishes. The most common benign skin diseases are discussed here. Although malignant diseases may initially appear as small facial blemishes, their treatment is beyond the scope of cosmetic surgery and will not be included.

MOLES (NEVI)

Perhaps the most common benign facial blemish is the pigmented *nevus*, commonly known as the mole (fig 4). The average person has fifteen to twenty moles, most of which have developed by puberty. Moles arise from *melanocytes*, the cells responsible for production of skin pigment. These growths commonly occur on the face and while many people want them removed, others find moles desirable, calling them "beauty marks."

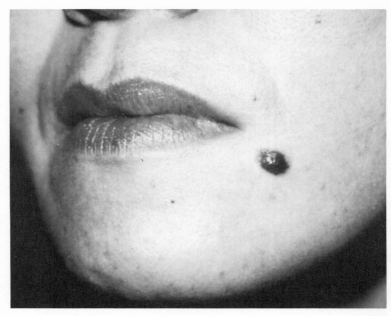

Fig. 4. Mole (Nevus).

Most moles are benign throughout life, but an occasional nevus develops into a skin cancer called *malignant melanoma.* The odds of such malignant transformation occurring in a given nevus are about 900,000 to 1. Many people, however, having heard or read about the deadly melanoma, want moles removed for this reason.

Certain danger signals frequently herald impending malignant transformation of a mole. These include a sudden change in shape, size, or color, or spread of pigmentation into the surrounding skin. A change in consistency (softness, firmness, etc.) or the surface texture of the mole, including scaliness, ulceration, crusting, oozing, or bleeding is another warning sign. Moles that itch or become tender or painful are also open to suspicion. Redness or swelling of the skin around a nevus is another reason for concern.

Moles exhibiting any of these characteristics should be removed without delay and submitted for microscopic examination. Facial nevi that are subjected to frequent irritation should also be excised. Other reasons for removing facial moles include wanting to eradicate a blemish, or the patient's fear of cancer.

Moles on the face can be removed by several of the techniques discussed. Surgical excision, placing the scar in a natural facial wrinkle, is a frequently utilized method. Some physicians recommend shave excision with electrodesiccation of the base. Excision using a skin punch is a third method of treatment. All excised nevi are submitted for microscopic examination to exclude the presence of malignancy.

SEBORRHEIC KERATOSIS

These growths, often called "senile warts" because of their irregular surface, commonly occur on the face (fig. 5). Many

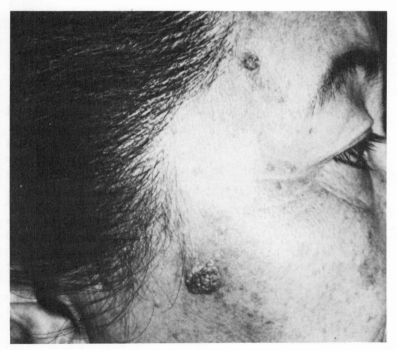

Fig. 5. Seborrheic keratosis.

people over fifty will develop *seborrheic keratoses*, which appear as flat, slightly elevated brown areas that gradually darken as they increase in thickness. These growths are completely benign and can be accurately diagnosed by a physician experienced in the treatment of skin disorders.

Seborrheic keratosis can be effectively removed by shave excision or curettage and electrodesiccation. Multiple growths are often removed by cryosurgery or the application of weak acids. These methods generally produce an imperceptible scar.

ACTINIC KERATOSIS

Actinic or *solar keratosis* is a localized, flat, or slightly elevated scaling patch of roughened skin that develops in many people who have a long history of sun exposure (fig 6). These areas represent a response of skin injured by sunlight and are more common in people with fair complexions. The color of actinic keratoses varies but most are red, yellowbrown, or gray. Occasionally such areas are flesh colored and their presence is noted only by feeling roughness when touching the skin.

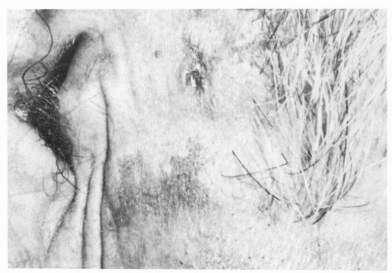

Fig. 6. Actinic keratosis.

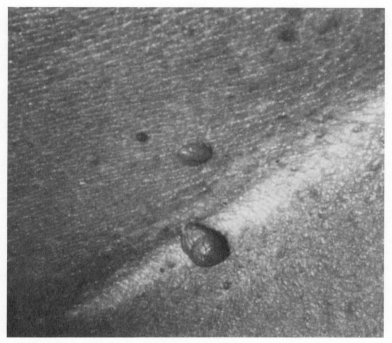

Fig. 7. Skin tag.

Unlike seborrheic keratoses, which are entirely benign, actinic keratoses may transform into malignancies and thus require treatment. Several forms of therapy are available including curettage, electrodesiccation, cryosurgery, and application of weak acids or phenol. These areas are frequently multiple and when they are, chemosurgery with topical application of the drug 5-flourouracil (5-FU) is generally recommended. An advantage of this form of treatment is that flesh-colored keratoses that are not visible are also eradicated. The treated areas become red and tender during therapy and exposure to sunlight should be avoided during this time.

SKIN TAGS

Skin tags are small, brown, fleshy growths that project from the skin surface (fig 7). These tags commonly occur on the neck and are occasionally found on the face. Small skin tags are effectively treated by application of weak acid solutions. Larger growths can be excised at their base with sharp scissors.

CYSTS

Small cysts arising beneath the surface of the skin are commonly found on the face. Such cysts usually develop from elements of the skin that become trapped below its surface. These elements continue to grow and slowly enlarge, forming a firm, smooth, rounded, and nontender mass that is easily felt. As such cysts are benign, most do not require treatment. Many patients, however, request their removal for cosmetic reasons. Occasionally a cyst becomes infected and must be surgically drained.

The preferred method of treating subcutaneous cysts is surgical excision, usually performed under local anesthesia in the surgeon's office. If the cyst is not completely excised, it may recur.

XANTHELASMA

Xanthelasma is a flat, yellowish plaque found on the upper and lower eyelids (fig 8). These plaques form as a consequence of deposition of cholesterol and other fat substances in the skin. Similar areas in other regions of the body are caused in association with elevated cholesterol and fat in the blood, but only about 50 percent of patients with xanthelasma exhibit increased blood levels of these substances.

TELANGIECTASIS

Telangiectasis is an abnormality of small blood vessels near the skin surface and is characterized by a small central blood vessel from which small, threadlike vessels radiate (fig. 9). The area can be blanched by gentle finger pressure but regains its color immediately upon release of pressure. Telangiectasis often develops spontaneously but is commonly associated with pregnancy. Patients with disorders of the liver frequently have multiple telangiectasis.

These areas are frequently eradicated by electrodesicca-

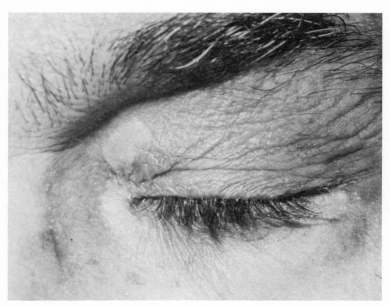

Fig. 8. Xanthelasma.

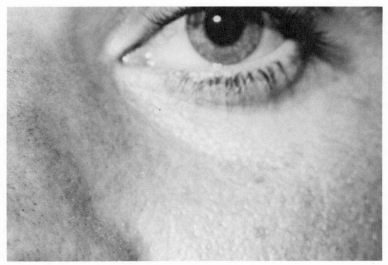

Fig. 9. Telangiectasia on nose.

tion or cryosurgery, but may recur. Occasionally, surgical excision is required for complete obliteration. These areas can often be hidden by cosmetics.

HEMANGIOMAS

Hemangiomas are formed by abnormal clusters of small blood vessels located just beneath the cutaneous surface. They impart a blue or red discoloration to the overlying skin. These areas usually develop before or shortly after birth and are thus commonly called birthmarks. Hemangiomas are classified according to the type of blood vessels that form them. They commonly occur on the face, forming blemishes of various sizes.

Some hemangiomas are elevated from the skin surface and have an irregular surface resembling a strawberry (fig. 10). Such strawberry hemangiomas usually disappear spon-

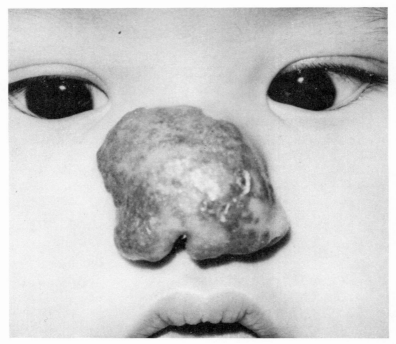

Fig. 10. Hemangioma.

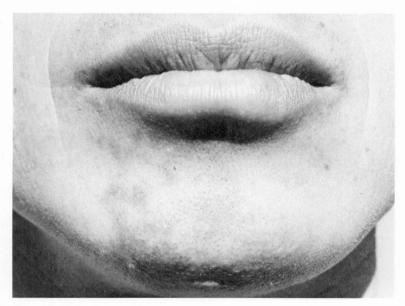

Fig. 11. Portwine stain.

taneously during early childhood and thus are rarely of concern to the cosmetic facial surgeon.

Most of the hemangiomas that persist into adulthood are composed of small capillary blood vessels located beneath the skin surface. These vessels impart a reddish-purple discoloration to the overlying skin and are commonly known as "portwine stains" (fig. 11). Facial hemangiomas can produce considerable disfigurement, and the cosmetic facial surgeon is frequently consulted about treatment.

Most portwine stains are large enough so that surgical removal would leave scars that might be more disfiguring than the hemangioma. Many hemangiomas can be effectively camouflaged by special cosmetic preparations, thus obviating the need for further treatment.

One form of treatment consists of tattooing the area of discoloration with a flesh-colored pigment. This results in improvement in many cases, but in others the pigment is gradually extruded from the skin and a blotchy appearance develops.

A recently developed method of treatment involves using a surgical laser beam to destroy the blood vessels of the hemangioma without damaging the overlying skin. Unfortunately, laser technology is relatively new and expensive and so is available in only a few medical centers. This method, however, will undoubtedly increase in popularity and if the preliminary encouraging reports of its usefulness are confirmed, laser treatment will offer new hope for those who have these disfiguring abnormalities.

9

Anatomy of the Face

A knowledge of the anatomy of the facial structure is helpful in understanding the various cosmetic surgical procedures used to modify these characteristics.

As in all other parts of the body, the basic superstructure or foundation of the face is the skeleton. This skeleton consists of bone in all areas except the eyes, ears, and lower half of the nose, where it is formed by cartilage or dense fibrous tissue.

Several large bones contribute to the facial skeleton (fig. 1). The forehead overlies the inferior portion of the frontal bone. The high point of the cheek is formed by the *zygomatic bone,* which articulates with the major bone of the midface—the *maxilla.* The upper teeth are imbedded in the maxilla and the small, paired nasal bones that provide skeletal support for the nasal bridge are attached to this bone. The skeleton of the lower jaw is formed by the mandible, from which the lower teeth arise. The lower border of the mandible forms the line of demarcation between the face and neck and its front surface is responsible for the chin prominence. The angle of the mandible can be felt just beneath the ear lobe.

A small bone located in the upper neck, the *hyoid* bone, is important in determining the angle between the chin and neck. In most people, this bone is located slightly above the

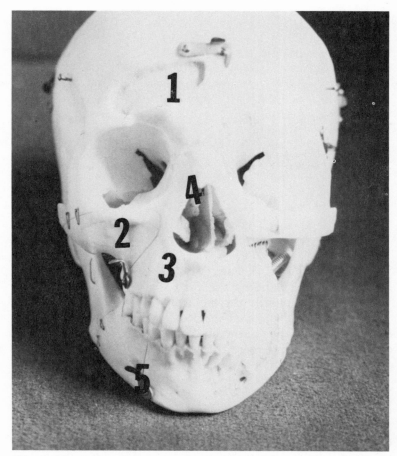

*Fig. 1. The facial skeleton (skull) composed of: (1) frontal bone,
(2) zygomatic bone, (3) maxilla, (4) nasal bone, (5) mandible.*

level of the chin and a sharp acute or right angle is formed at
this junction. People with low-placed hyoid bones show an
obtuse angle at this junction, producing webbing that may
contribute to the appearance of a double chin (fig. 2).

The lower half of the nasal skeleton is composed of cartilage. The lower lateral cartilage, which assumes an archlike
configuration around the nostrils, forms the framework of the
tip. The upper lateral cartilage bridges the gap between the

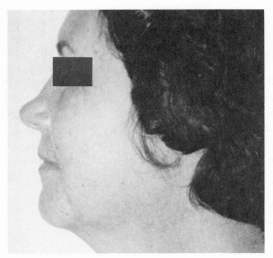

Fig. 2. Double chin secondary to low placement of hyoid.

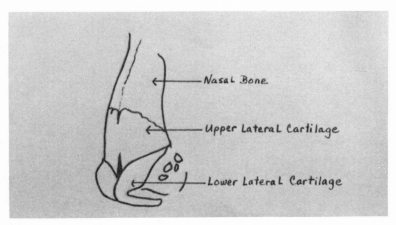

Fig. 3. The nasal skeleton.

nasal bones and lower lateral cartilages, completing the nasal skeleton (fig. 3). The skeletal support of the ear and eyelids is formed entirely by cartilage.

The teeth, though not actually a part of the skeleton, are important in the configuration of the lower part of the face. The position of the teeth influences the posture of the upper and lower lip. The loss of teeth is accompanied by degeneration of the portions of the maxilla and mandible into which they are inserted, causing a decrease in the vertical dimension of the teeth and consequent abnormalities of the lips. This topic is discussed in detail in chapter 16. Variations in the facial skeleton are mainly responsible for the large variations in facial characteristics. Although the characteristics of facial skeleton are controlled largely by heredity, they are subject to modification by injury, disease, and, to some extent, by surgery.

The facial skin drapes over the skeleton, producing the fine elements of the facial features. This skin varies in thickness in different areas. It is thin over the eyelids, ears, and upper half of the nose, and thick over the forehead, cheeks, and lower half of the nose.

Skin is composed of a thin outer layer, the *epidermis*, and a thicker lower layer of *dermis*. The epidermis is equipped with appendages of two types—hair follicles, from which hair grows, and glands, which produce secretions of various types (sweat glands, sebaceous glands, etc.). The lower layer of the epidermis contains cells called *melanocytes*, which produce pigment (melanin) that is responsible for the color of the skin.

Skin texture is largely determined by the characteristics of the dermis, including its thickness, degree of hydration and elasticity.

Tissue lying beneath the dermis is called subcutaneous tissue and consists mainly of fat. The thickness of this fat varies from person to person and from area to area. Its thickness also varies with fluctuations in body weight and tends to decrease with age. It is one of the factors responsible for the aging of the face.

Large deposits of fat tend to accumulate in two areas of the face. Accumulation in the cheek area is called the *buccal fat pad*, and the deposit beneath the chin is called the *submental fat pad*. The buccal fat pad tends to decrease in size during aging, resulting in a hollow appearance in the cheeks. The submental fat pads, however, tend to increase in size with age, contributing to the formation of the double chin.

The blood supply to the facial skin is located between the dermis and subcutaneous tissue, and thus in the face-lift procedure, a small amount of fat is left on the facial skin (see chapter 11).

The *parotid gland*, one of the major salivary glands, lies beneath the facial skin in front of the ear and just behind the buccal fat pad. It contributes to the fullness of the face.

The muscles of facial expression lie beneath the subcutaneous tissue (fig. 4). These muscles are unique in that they are the only muscles of the body that insert into the skin. Because of these insertions, contraction of these muscles alters the contour of the facial skin, giving rise to the various forms of human expression. The activity of these muscles is also responsible for many of the facial wrinkles that occur with aging—wrinkles always developing in a direction perpendicular to the direction of muscle contraction.

The muscles of facial expression can be divided into five

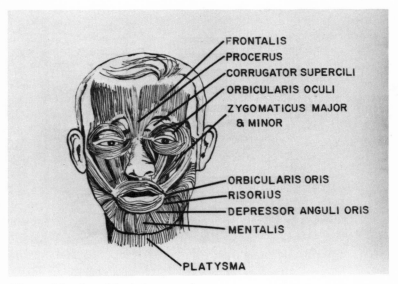

Fig. 4. Muscles of facial expression.

major groups according to the areas in which they are located.

The major muscle of the forehead is the *frontalis*. Its fibers are aligned vertically. Contraction of this muscle tenses the forehead skin and elevates the eyebrows. The activity of this muscle is responsible for the horizontal frown lines of the forehead that appear in mid adulthood (fig. 5).

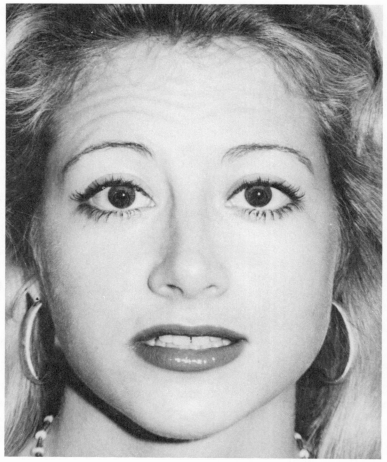

Fig. 5. Horizontal frown lines produced by activity of the frontalis muscle.

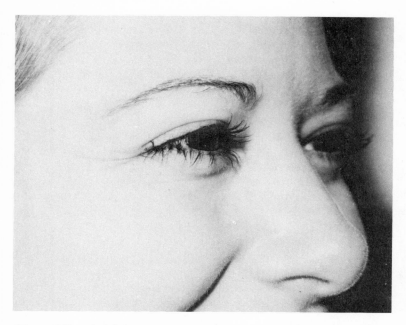

Fig. 6. "Crow's-feet" or "laugh lines" produced by the orbicularis oculi muscle.

The major muscle underlying the eyelids is the *orbicularis oculi*. The fibers of this muscle are arranged in a circular fashion around the eye. Contraction of the portion of this muscle under the upper lid results in closure of the eye. Contraction of the entire muscle draws the brow downward and the lower lid and adjacent part of the cheek upward as in a squint. Activity of this muscle is responsible for the "crow's-feet" or "laugh lines" found at the outer edge of the eyelids (fig. 6).

The *corrugator supercilii* are small but relatively powerful muscles that insert into the eyebrow. Contraction of this muscle pulls the brow toward the center of the face and is responsible for producing the vertical frown lines that develop above the root of the nose during aging (fig. 7).

Several small muscles of facial expression lie beneath the nasal skin. The *nasalis* muscle courses across the nose just

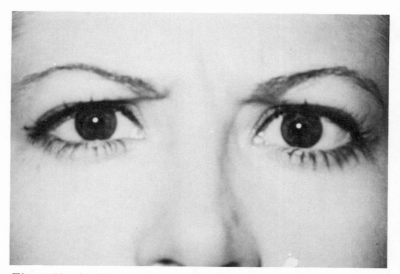

Fig. 7. Vertical frown lines produced by the corrugator supercilii muscles.

above the tip and is thought to compress the nostrils. Two small muscles, the *dilator nares*, counteract the nasalis by dilating the nostrils. The *depressor septi* inserts beneath the base of the nose, and contraction pulls the tip toward the lip and tends to narrow the nostrils. The action of this muscle may produce transverse wrinkles beneath the base of the nose. The *procerus* muscle lies beneath the skin of the nasal root and its contraction pulls the skin of this area down, producing transverse wrinkling at the nasal root.

Muscles of facial expression related to the mouth comprise the largest group. A large muscle, the *orbicularis oris*, surrounds the mouth in a circular fashion in somewhat the same way that the orbicularis oculi surrounds the eye. Contraction results in closure of the lips and pulls them against the teeth, or produces a pursing posture (fig. 8).

The *zygomatic major* and *minor* muscles, commonly known as the "smile" muscles, insert into the skin of the upper lip (fig 9). Contraction of these muscles elevates the corner of the mouth, producing a smile. The activity of these muscles con-

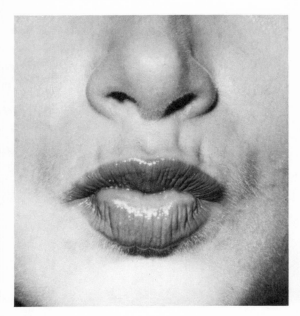

Fig. 8. Pursing of the lips produced by the orbicularis oris muscle.

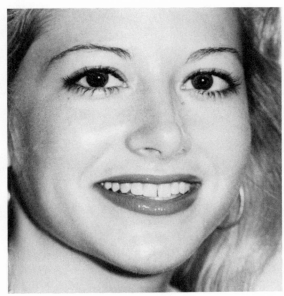

Fig. 9. Smile produced by the zygomatic major and minor muscles.

tributes to producing the deep crease that may develop between the nose and corners of the mouth (nasolabial fold).

The *risorius* muscle inserts into the corner of the mouth and its contraction draws the mouth laterally as occurs during a "smirk" (fig. 10). Such contractions may also contribute to development of the nasolabial fold.

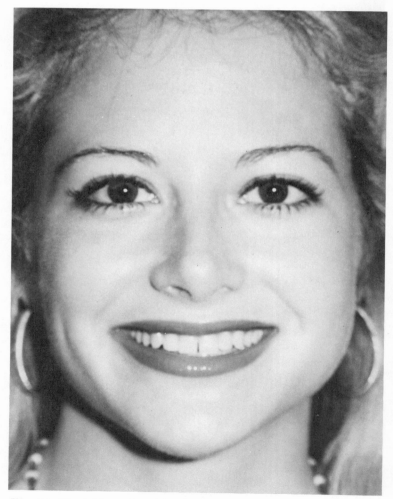

Fig. 10. "Smirk" produced by the risorius muscle.

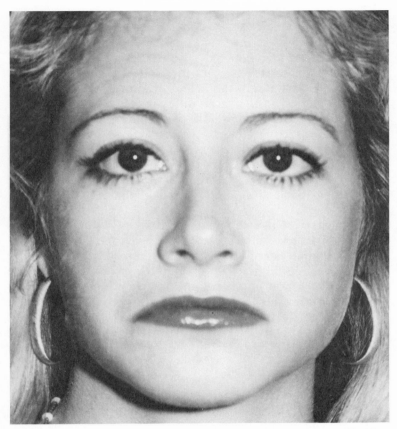

Fig. 11. "Pouting" produced by the depressor labii and anguli oris muscles.

Several other muscles insert into the upper lip and assist in drawing it upward. These are the *levator labii superioris* and the *levator anguli oris.* The *levator labii superioris alaeque nasi* also elevates the base of the nose and produces dilation of the nostrils.

Two muscles insert into the skin of the lower lip, the *depressor labii inferioris* and *depressor anguli oris.* Contraction of these muscles draws the lower lip downward (fig. 11).

The *mentalis* muscle inserts into the skin of the chin and draws this skin upward, aiding in puckering the lip.

The *buccinator* is a large muscle beneath the skin of the cheek. Contraction draws the cheek inward against the cheek. This muscle is rarely involved in facial expression, but functions mainly during chewing.

Three small muscles insert into the skin beneath the attachments of the ear to the face. These muscles are usually poorly developed and have no function, but they are responsible for the ability to wiggle the ear, which some people have.

A muscle of expression, the *platysma*, also lies beneath the skin of the neck. This muscle is also poorly developed in many people. Its contraction tenses the skin of the neck and when well-developed, it may contribute to formation of the bridle-like vertical bands frequently noted in the aging neck (fig. 12).

The degree of development and activity of the muscles of facial expression varies significantly from person to person. A major cranial nerve—appropriately named the facial nerve—is responsible for the nerve supply to these muscles. The complexity of this nerve supply, which is under conscious control, is responsible for the remarkable variability of facial expression characteristic of the human face. Unfortunately, it is likely that this animation of the face is partly responsible for the signs of aging (see chapter 10).

Brief Anatomic Details of Facial Structures

Eyes: The eyes are located in a bony cavity called the orbit, which protects the globe (eyeball) housing the sensory organ of sight. The eyelid skeleton consists of dense fibrous tissue called the *tarsal plates*. Further details of the anatomy of the eye are found in the chapter on blepharoplasty.

Ears: The ears project from the sides of the face with varying degrees of prominence (see chapter 17). The superior attachment of the ear (also called the *auricle* or *pinna*) is at the level of the eye, and the inferior attachment of the lobe approximates the level of the base of the nose (fig. 13). The skeleton of the auricle is formed by cartilage that in turn forms the delicate convolutions that give the ear its thin intricate shape (see chapter 17). The skin of the ear is thin and adheres tightly to the cartilage. An external opening or *meatus* leads into the

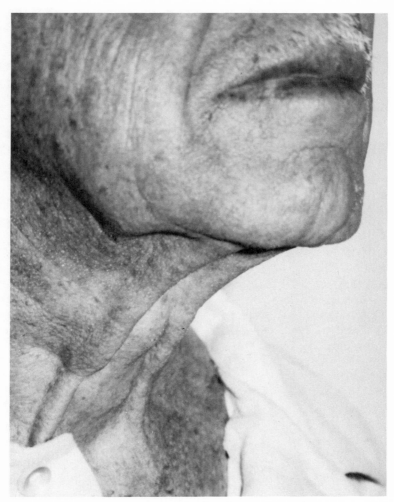

Fig. 12. Neck bands produced by the platysma muscle.

external auditory canal, at the end of which is the tympanic membrane or eardrum.

Mouth: The mouth, which serves as the point of entry to the digestive system, is located approximately one-third of the distance between the base of the nose and the chin. It is

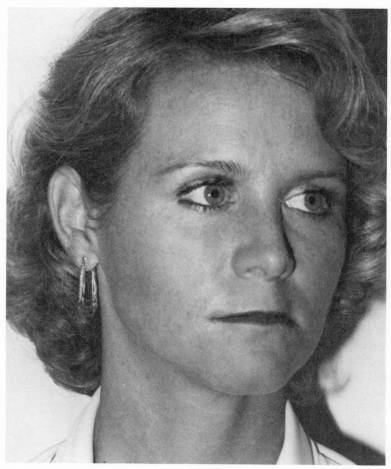

Fig. 13. Attachment of the ear at the level of the eye and the base of the nose.

bounded by the upper and lower lips, which are muscular structures covered with thin, transparent *epithelium* called the vermilion, which transmits the reddish hue of the underlying blood vessels (fig. 14). The junction of the vermilion with the facial skin is called the *mucocutaneous junction* and is normally a sharp line of demarcation. The center of the upper lip forms a prominence called the tubercle. Above the

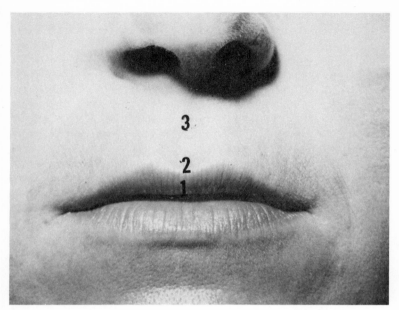

Fig. 14. The lip: (1) tubercle, (2) "Cupid's bow," (3) philtrum.

tubercle, the mucocutaneous junction courses in M-shaped fashion to form the "Cupid's bow." The *philtrum* extends from this bow to the base of the nose. The basic function of the lips is to provide a seal for the mouth during chewing. Other than the eyes, the lips are the most expressive structures of the face.

Nose: The nose projects from the face and exhibits great variation in size and configuration. The thickness of the nasal skin varies in different parts of the nose. Over the tip and lower third, the skin and subcutaneous tissue is thick and well-endowed with glands that produce greasy sebaceous material. The skin and subcutaneous tissue gradually thins over the upper cartilaginous and bony skeletons. The skin then increases in thickness over the nasal bridge and is relatively thick where it joins the forehead. The thickness and consistency of the nasal skin shows considerable individual, sexual, and racial variations.

The great variation between these features of the human face results in an infinite array of facial characteristics. Indeed, it is certainly true that no two faces are exactly alike. The desirable attributes of each facial structure and their relationships, which combine to form our perception of harmony and beauty, are discussed in chapter 9. These features are further discussed in the chapters describing surgical modification of individual structures.

10

The Aging Face

While aging is associated with wisdom and maturity in many cultures, contemporary Western society places a premium on a youthful, vibrant appearance. To an increasing extent, conformity to this standard is important to a person's psychological, social, and economic success.

As the birth rate declines and modern medicine continues its conquest of disease, an increasing percentage of the population will reach old age, intensifying the current demand for measures to counteract the manifestations of aging. Throughout history, man has searched for methods to turn back the biologic clock, but until techniques of cosmetic surgery were developed, this search had been fruitless.

Because the face shows age earlier and to a greater extent than other parts of the body, interest in facial rejuvenation has been in the forefront of progress in cosmetic surgery. In the past, surgical procedures designed to combat facial aging were available only to the affluent, but cosmetic facial surgery is now within the reach of most who want it.

While cosmetic facial surgery may appear to offer much with regard to turning back the clock, its techniques should be placed in proper perspective. Cosmetic surgery merely alters the superficial appearance of the face (thus the designation "cosmetic") and provides no relief for the cellular and biochemical mechanisms that are the true causes of aging. Comprehension and alteration of these processes are goals for future generations.

Theories of Aging

Many theories have been proposed to explain aging, but as none are in complete agreement with all available data, the exact reasons remain uncertain.

Perhaps the most simplistic theory holds that in later years, the metabolic machinery of the body becomes gradually exhausted and finally wears out, much as any other machine. One variant of this theory is that this cellular exhaustion is the result of the gradual accumulation of oxidants and other deleterious products of metabolism. While this may be true, these theories offer no adequate explanation of the causes of these processes.

Some of the most popular theories of aging relate to genetic or hereditary causes. One theory is that from the beginning each cell is genetically endowed with a programmed message dictating its course of aging and its time of natural death. A related theory states that genetic mutations, which are known to occur periodically during the growth and division of a cell, may result in changes that adversely affect the organism.

A third variant, the auto-immune theory, holds that mutations in cells that are responsible for producing antibodies result in formation of abnormal antibodies that attack the cells of the organism and result in their destruction. Such mutations could occur as a result of many factors, including exposure to radiation, noxious chemicals, or viral infection.

Regardless of the veracity of the various genetic theories of aging, the modifying effects of environment on heredity are well-known. There is no reason to suspect that this relationship would not also operate in conjunction with the factors described in the genetic theories. Such environmental factors, known to influence aging of the face, are discussed below.

Environmental Causes of Facial Aging

By far the most important environmental factor in facial aging is exposure to sunlight. Although a suntan is almost universally considered a sign of vitality and good health, the cumulative effect of exposure to the sun's rays is the most potent factor in aging of the skin. Microscopic examination of skin from the face and from the unexposed areas of the body of people frequently exposed to the sun consistently shows marked degeneration of the structural components of the facial skin and no significant degeneration of unexposed skin. The early facial aging of farmers, sailors, cowboys, and other people whose work continually exposes them to the sun graphically demonstrates this point. Reflection from sand and snow intensifies the effects of the sun.

The natural color of the skin significantly modifies the response of the skin to sunlight. The pigment *melanin*, which is present in increased amounts in the dark-skinned races, offers considerable protection against these damaging effects. This accounts for the relatively young appearances of many old members of the black and brown races.

The damage sunlight does to the skin is not immediately apparent to the sunworshipper. Microscopic abnormalities accumulate only to become noticeable many years later. Thus despite repeated warnings, people remain oblivious to the consequences of frequent sunning. In addition to accelerating aging, exposure to the sun is a potent factor in the development of skin cancer.

Fortunately, the patient individual can acquire a suntan without needless exposure to the damaging rays of the sun. These destructive rays lie within the spectrum (290-310 μ), which is responsible for sunburn. Sunscreens effectively block this spectrum while permitting penetration of the tanning rays that occupy the long ultraviolet spectrum. The most effective of these sunscreens are para-aminobenzoic acid (PABA) and benzophenones, both of which are available in commercial products. The skin-damaging rays of the sun are less intense in the Northern hemisphere before 10:00 A.M. or after 3:00 P.M. A wide-brimmed hat is also effective in protecting the facial skin during these hours. Exposure to the wind and other elements also accelerates deterioration of the facial skin.

Weight gain stretches the skin and ruptures its attachments to the underlying facial tissue. It predisposes to sagging and redundancy if the weight is subsequently lost. Severe illnesses or chronic nutritional deficiencies may also accelerate aging of the skin.

All of these environmental factors act in concert with hereditary endowment to determine the rate and extent of facial aging in each person.

Microscopic Changes in Aging Skin

All visible changes in the aging skin are related to basic alterations in cellular structure visible only under the microscope. The first signs of degeneration, of course, develop long before the signs of aging are apparent on the skin's surface. Characteristic changes occur in both layers of the skin—the *epidermis* and underlying *dermis*.

The epidermis, or outer layer, gradually decreases in thickness with aging. The melanin-producing cells decrease in number, resulting in less production of pigment for protection of the skin against ultraviolet radiation. In some areas, these cells accumulate in increased numbers producing the familiar "age spots" called *lentigines*.

The dermis, the characteristics of which determine the thickness and texture of skin, undergoes more significant changes during aging. Fibrous supporting tissue in this layer— which is composed of fibers of *collagen*, the main structural protein of the body—thickens and becomes less extensible, resulting in decreased elasticity of the skin. Elastic fibers in the dermis also gradually deteriorate, contributing to this decreased elasticity. Elastic fiber degeneration is markedly accelerated in areas exposed to the sun.

The water content of the dermis gradually declines, accounting for the leathery toughness of aging skin as compared to the softness and resilience of youthful skin. The subcutaneous fat also becomes less thick during aging and its fibrous connections with underlying tissue become attenuated, resulting in some loss of support.

As a result of these degenerative changes, aging skin is characteristically sallow, thin, tough, and wrinkled in contrast to the pink, smooth, thick, resilient skin of youth. Areas of increased and decreased pigmentation are common because of the changes in melanin.

Characteristics of Aging Facial Skin

In addition to these general changes in skin texture, aging of the face is characterized by sagging, wrinkling, and the development of areas of hollowness. A hollow appearance in the cheeks results from absorption of fat deposits (buccal fat pad) underlying this area. Hollowness often occurs in the temple areas as well as around the eyelid.

Sagging occurs from the effects of gravity on redundant skin. Several factors other than the general loss of elasticity contribute to redundancy of the facial skin. The entire skull tends to decrease in size during aging. In association with gradual absorption of the subcutaneous fat tissue, this results in a smaller surface area for skin to cover. As the skin envelope is of fixed size, or is slightly increased in size secondary to loss of elasticity, redundancy and sagging are inevitable. Redundancy of the lips is accentuated by loss of the teeth, which is accompanied by absorption of portions of the jaws, resulting in a shortening of the skeletal structure of the middle of the face.

Skin wrinkles can be divided into three major groups. Lines at the junction of facial structures—such as the junction of the ear and face, or cheek and nose—are called contour lines. These wrinkles are not a manifestation of aging but are usually accentuated with age.

The lines of relaxed skin tension (RSTL), also called dynamic wrinkles, are caused by contraction of facial muscles that are attached directly to the skin. These wrinkles are formed at right angles to the long axis of muscle contraction and are illustrated in figure 1. (A detailed discussion of the muscles of facial expression is found in chapter 9.)

The third major group of facial wrinkles are called dependency or gravitational lines. They are caused by the ef-

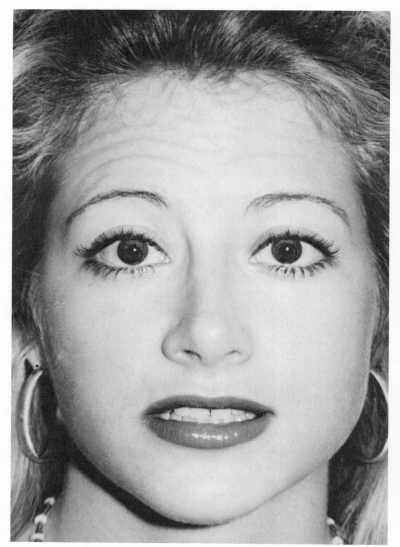

Fig. 1. Horizontal forehead wrinkles.

fects of gravity on redundant skin. Characteristic gravitational lines are illustrated in figure 2.

Temporal Patterns of Facial Aging

Sagging and wrinkling of the facial skin, although varying tremendously from person to person because of both hereditary and environmental factors, generally follows a characteristic temporal pattern. The first facial wrinkles to develop are horizontal furrows in the forehead that may occur in the early twenties and are a result of contraction of the underlying *frontalis* muscle (fig. 3).

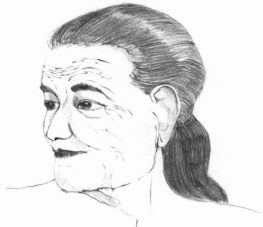

Fig. 2. Gravitational lines.

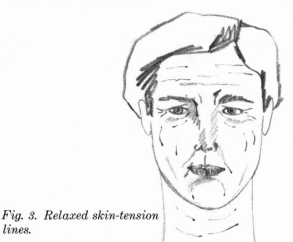

Fig. 3. Relaxed skin-tension lines.

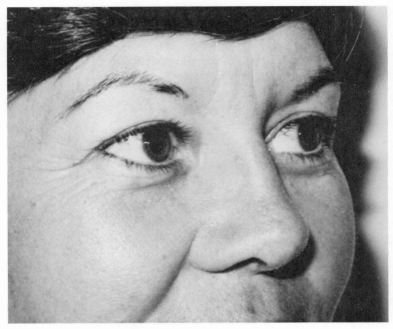

Fig. 4. "Crow's-feet" or "laugh lines."

At thirty, sagging of the upper lids begins and is accompanied by the appearance of "laugh lines" or "crow's-feet" around the outside corner of the eyes (fig. 4).

During the forties, the laugh lines deepen and the skin of the upper lid becomes increasingly redundant. A sharp line of demarcation between the lower eyelid and cheek is often apparent. It may be accentuated by puffiness of the lower lid secondary to laxity of periorbital fat or intermittent accumulation of fluid (fig. 5).

The *nasolabial folds* become more prominent during this decade, and sagging of redundant skin over the lower jaw starts to form the jowl (fig. 6).

At fifty, the outside corner of the eye begins to droop, resulting in a tired or sad appearance (fig. 7). The nasolabial fold becomes deeper and may continue toward the chin as a deep furrow (fig. 6). The skin of the neck begins to sag, and an

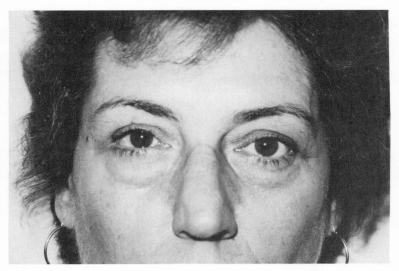

Fig. 5. Redundancy of upper eyelid skin and puffiness of lower eyelids.

Fig. 6. Jowl formation with fat accumulation in neck producing double chin.

Fig. 7. Downward slant of eyes, deep nasolabial folds continuing towards chin.

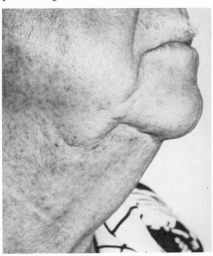

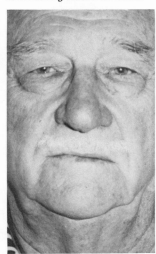

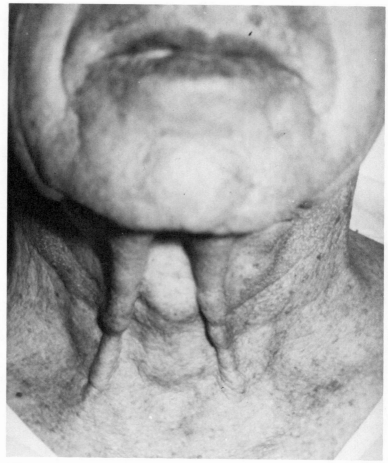

Fig. 8. Bridlelike neck bands and laxity of skin produces "turkey gobbler" neck.

accumulation of fat beneath the chin may produce a double chin (fig. 7).

Activity of the *platysma* muscle in the neck often contributes to formation of bridlelike bands that course in a vertical direction, contributing to creating the "turkey gobbler" neck (fig. 8).

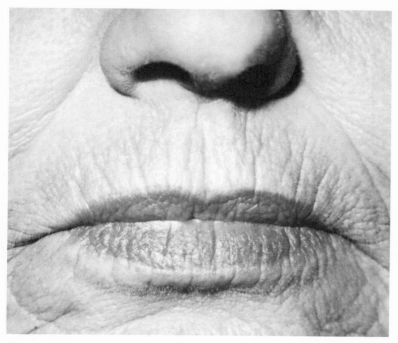

Fig. 9. Vertical lip wrinkles.

Vertical wrinkling of the lips may also occur between fifty and sixty (fig. 9). These wrinkles are caused by contraction of the underlying *orbicularis oris* muscle and may be more prominent in people who constantly purse their lips while smoking.

During the late fifties and sixties, absorption of fat tissue in the cheeks and temples gives these areas a hollow appearance. Absorption of fat beneath the eyelids may also produce a hollow or sunken appearance of the eyes.

The tip of the nose may also begin to droop during this period. Descent of the tip makes the nasal bridge more prominent and may produce a frank nasal hump. Drooping of the tip may give the nose a "hooked" appearance. In later years all these changes intensify. Multiple, fine facial wrinkles often appear, resulting in development of the "prune face" (fig. 10).

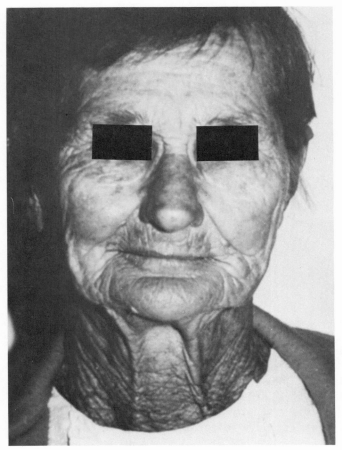

Fig. 10. Hollowing of cheeks and temples and finely etched wrinkles produce "prune face."

Further discussion of the changes in various facial structures that are caused by aging is found in the chapters on cosmetic surgical procedures relative to those areas.

11

The Face-Lift Operation

To a large segment of the population, cosmetic facial surgery is almost synonomous with the face-lift operation. The desire to maintain a youthful appearance has characterized man throughout recorded history, and for many people, the face-lift procedure is the epitome of this desire. This operation has been glamorized by the press, television, and the motion picture industry to such an extent that it is surrounded by an air of mysticism. In some circles, the face-lift is a status symbol.

Such glamorization, of course, frequently results in superficial understanding and misconceptions, and this is certainly true in the case of the face-lift operation. As in any surgical procedure, optimum results can be obtained only after careful preoperative assessment and selection of proper candidates. Not all people can receive the same benefit from a surgical face-lift.

The purpose of face-lift surgery is to remove redundant, sagging skin from the face and neck and to reduce wrinkling associated with aging. Actually, repositioning or redraping of skin over the facial bones is just as important in achieving the desired result as is removal of skin.

Several medical terms are used to describe the face-lift operation. The most common, *rhytidectomy*, is derived from *rhytis*—wrinkle; and *ectomy*—removal or excision. Other common terms include *rhytidoplasty* (*plasty*—alteration of shape or form), *meloplasty* (*melo*—cheek) and *prosopexy* (*pros*—face; *pexy*—lifting or elevation).

Causes of facial aging are discussed in chapter 10. Reviewing this material may be of help in understanding the description of the face-lift operation.

History of the Surgical Face-Lift

Although the exact origins of the face-lift operation are uncertain, such surgery was being performed in Europe during the early twentieth century. As cosmetic surgery was not sanctioned then, the face-lift and other cosmetic operations were performed in secrecy and surgical techniques were not published in medical journals or discussed at medical meetings.

Improvement in techniques of plastic surgery was spurred by the need to treat extensive war wounds, advances in pre- and postoperative care, and control of infection. Changes in the attitude of modern society toward cosmetic surgery, allowed the application of medical and surgical technology to the area of cosmetic surgery. The improved general health and affluence of those who are candidates for face-lift surgery has also enhanced its popularity.

The face-lift operation has undergone many refinements and modifications since its inception, and the properly screened patient can expect a satisfactory result when treated by a qualified surgeon. The popularity of the operation will undoubtedly increase as the percentage of older people in the population continues to increase.

Reasons for Face-Lift Surgery

As discussed in chapter 1, there are several valid reasons for wanting to undergo cosmetic facial surgery. Besides the obvious wish to regain a youthful appearance, economic, social, and psychologic reasons may be strong. In modern society, a premium is placed on presenting a vigorous and youthful appearance. An improved appearance may bolster sagging self-esteem and supply a fresh charge of emotional energy that gives a person a new outlook on life.

Although most people who want face-lift surgery are women, a significant percentage of requests now come from men. As the economic, social, and psychologic benefits from cosmetic facial surgery become more apparent, it is probable that even more men will develop an interest in this procedure.

Alternatives to the Surgical Face-Lift

From time to time, enthusiastic advertisements extol various methods of facial rejuvenation without surgery. Such methods include facial massage, facial exercises, and various creams, lotions, and ointments for application to the face. One manufacturer has even promoted a device for facial suction.

While the various facial preparations may be of some benefit (functioning by rehydrating the skin) such benefit is only temporary and is certainly not of the magnitude offered by the face-lift operation. Other facial creams contain mild skin irritants that cause some swelling that temporarily hides fine wrinkles. The reddish facial tint produced by this skin irritation may also suggest a healthy, vibrant look. The facial suction device may produce temporary improvement in a similar way.

The value of facial exercises or massage in rejuvenating the aging face is controversial at best. Most cosmetic facial surgeons feel that these methods may actually enhance or accelerate facial wrinkling because so many skin wrinkles characteristic of the aging face are caused by activity of the facial muscles, which pull, stretch, and crease the overlying skin (see chapter 9).

What a Face-Lift Can and Cannot Do

The face-lift operation is most effective in eliminating sagging, redundant skin around the jowls and upper neck. While some improvement in the deep creases extending from the base of the nose to the corner of the mouth (nasolabial

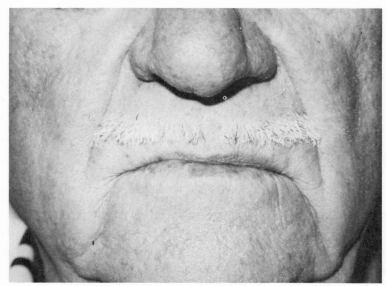

Fig. 1. Deep nasolabial folds extending from mouth towards chin (labiomental folds).

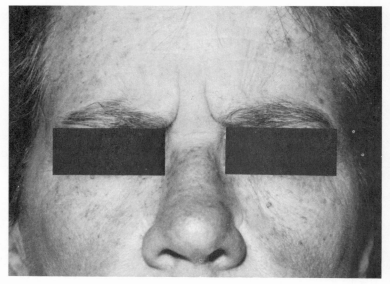

Fig. 2. Vertical (glabellar) "frown lines."

folds, fig. 1) can be expected, deep creases require ancillary measures for satisfactory effacement. Extensions of the nasolabial folds from the corner of the mouth toward the chin may also gain minimal benefit from face-lift surgery. Similarly, deep skin creases between the eye and root of the nose "frown lines" (fig. 2) and deep creases in the forehead are not corrected by the standard face-lift operation.

Wrinkled and sagging eyelid skin is not amenable to correction by the face-lift. It requires the *blepharoplasty* procedure for improvement (see chapter 12). This operation is often performed in conjunction with the face-lift.

Fine vertical wrinkles around the lips (fig. 3) also require other corrective procedures, most commonly chemosurgery (see chapter 19) or dermabrasion (see chapter 20). Fine wrinkles in other areas of the face also require chemosurgery or dermabrasion.

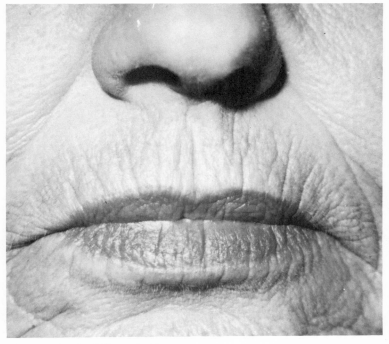

Fig. 3. Vertical lip wrinkles.

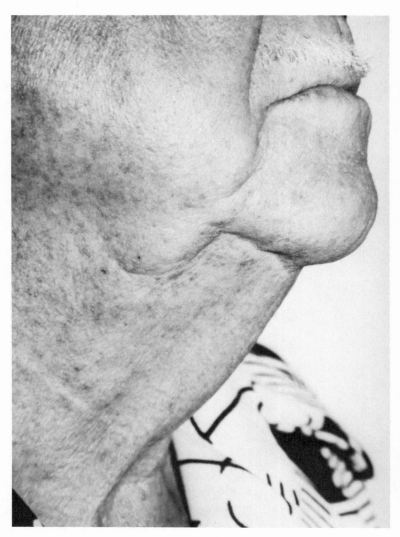

Fig. 4. Double chin.

The double chin (fig. 4) and the firm bridlelike bands that may be present in the anterior neck (fig. 5) are not corrected by the standard face-lift operation. These deformities necessitate other measures. Sagging or webbing of the upper neck

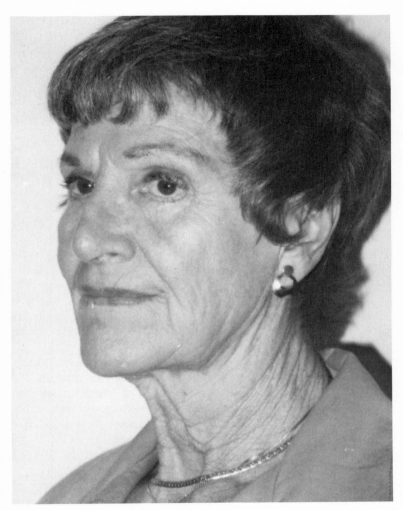

Fig. 5. Bridlelike bands in neck.

resulting from a low laryngeal skeleton cannot be modified by face-lift operation. Such webbing is usually hereditary and present since early adulthood.

It is important to realize that the face-lift cannot improve the quality and texture of the skin. Thin, poorly hydrated, weather-beaten, or leathery skin etched with multiple, fine wrinkles (which in extreme cases produce a shriveled, prune-like appearance) cannot be transformed into the smooth, resilient skin of youth by this or any other available technique, although chemosurgery may offer improvement in some cases.

Selection of Candidates
for the Face-Lift Operation

Prospective face-lift patients are carefully screened by the cosmetic facial surgeon. The structure of the facial skeleton is particularly important in that it forms the foundation over which the facial skin is draped after surgery. Ideal candidates have high cheekbones, a prominent mandible (jaw), a firm chin, and a neckline that exhibits a sharp chin-neck angle (fig. 6). While the absence of these skeletal characteristics does not mean a person should not have the operation, the surgical result may be compromised, and this must be carefully discussed with the patient.

Ideal candidates exhibit resilient, firm, smooth, and well hydrated skin. Face-lift surgery does not improve fine wrinkling and patients with this problem must understand this limitation.

The ideal candidate is in his early or mid-forties and exhibits early or moderately advanced degrees of facial aging, such as jowl formation or sagging skin in the anterior portion of the neck. Patients in this age group are also more likely to have the skin qualities discussed above. Such a candidate has rarely developed the deep nasolabial folds and other advanced creases described under the heading "What a Face-Lift Can and Cannot Do."

An ideal candidate is relatively thin with a stable weight pattern or a history of recent dietary weight loss. The results of face-lift surgery are frequently compromised by fluctuations in weight, as the skin stretches during the gain phase causing recurrent sagging when the excess weight is lost.

Just as important as physical characteristics in the screening of people for the face-lift operation are psychological or emotional factors. One of the most important requirements is that the patient's expectations be reasonable and realistic. As previously noted, glamorization of this procedure has re-

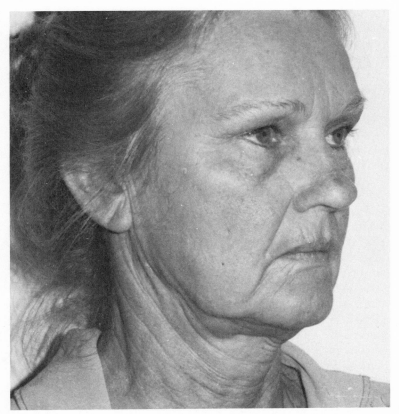

Fig. 6. Ideal candidate for face-lift operation. Note prominent cheekbone and jawline with sharp chin–neck angle and absence of fine skin wrinkling.

sulted in many misconceptions. For this reason, the surgeon is careful to stress the limitations of the procedure to the prospective patient, particularly the candidate who has physical defects that cannot be corrected by surgery. Such frank discussions can do much to minimize patient disappointment and dissatisfaction in the postoperative period. (This stance is particularly important for medicolegal reasons.)

The surgeon must also be satisfied with the prospective patient's motive for surgery. There are many acceptable motives for face-lift surgery (see chapter 1, Reasons for Seeking

Cosmetic Facial Surgery). Occasionally a patient may be asked to undergo psychological or psychiatric evaluation before acceptance for surgery if the surgeon does not feel comfortable with the patient's motives.

Candidates for the face-lift operation must be in good general health. Such surgery is not justified if it would jeopardize the physical or mental wellbeing of the patient. While this does not necessarily exclude patients with chronic medical disorders, these conditions must be satisfactorily controlled before surgery.

Preparation for Face-Lift Surgery

Preparation for the face-lift operation begins with final acceptance of the candidate for surgery. The patient is carefully counselled about important details of the surgical procedure and postoperative period. The expectations of the surgeon concerning the conduct of the patient during the critical postoperative healing period are thoroughly discussed.

Medical photographs are obtained and reviewed with the patient. Particular emphasis is placed on the areas to be corrected and on associated defects and asymmetries that the patient may not have noticed. Failure to point out such areas before the operation may result in disappointment during the postoperative period when the entire face is carefully scrutinized.

The location and extent of the scars that will result from the operation are discussed and the process of scar maturation is described. Possible complications are explained and the patient is encouraged to ask questions about things he does not fully understand. An informed consent agreement, giving the surgeon permission to perform the operation, is then executed.

Recent studies of informed consent agreements have shown that surgical patients remember only 20 to 30 percent of the information discussed during preoperative interviews. For this reason, some surgeons tape-record counselling sessions. Literature reviewing the material discussed during preoperative interviews may also be given to the patient.

Fees for face-lift surgery are usually paid in advance and

a member of the surgeon's office staff discusses them with the patient prior to final scheduling of surgery (see chapter 1).

Final Preoperative Instructions

The patient is told to avoid the use of aspirin or other medications that may interfere with the clotting mechanism of the blood. The surgeon will ask the patient for a list of the medications he usually takes in order to make this determination. An attempt will be made to avoid scheduling the operation during the menstrual period as it may cause increased operative bleeding. The patient may be instructed to wash the face and shampoo for several days before surgery in order to reduce the chances of postoperative infection.

Hospital Admission

If the face-lift is to be performed in a hospital, the patient is generally admitted on the evening before surgery for physical examination and to undergo laboratory procedures. Many surgeons perform the face-lift operation in outpatient surgical facilities, in which case the patient enters on the day of surgery and is discharged several hours after it. If the operation is scheduled this way, the patient is told to avoid solid food for six to eight hours before surgery. This minimizes the chance of vomiting.

Generally the hair is not shaved before face-lift surgery, but it may be clipped in the area where incisions are planned. This can be done on the evening before surgery or in the operating room.

Preoperative Medication Given

Sedatives in the form of pills and injections are administered one to two hours before surgery. On arrival in the operating room, an intravenous infusion is started through which more sedatives can be given if necessary. Then instruments that monitor cardiac activity and blood pressure are connected.

Anesthesia for the Face-Lift Operation

Most face-lifts are performed under local anesthesia (see chapter 6). If this is the case, the anesthetic solution is infiltrated into the operative field with a small hypodermic needle. If the operation is to be performed under general anesthesia, an anesthesiologist will be present to administer the anesthetics.

The Face-Lift Operation

First the operative field is cleaned with antiseptic solution, then sterile drapes are placed around the operative field to prevent its contamination.

The incision lines are then carefully outlined on the face with a marking pen. The usual face-lift incision (fig. 7) begins in the natural crease at the junction of the ear and face. At the ear lobe, the incision continues posteriorly, ascending in the crease between the ear and mastoid. At the level of the ear canal, the incision curves backward and extends into the hairline. The upper portion of the incision extends into the temporal hair, generally curving slightly forward. The surgeon may modify this basic incision depending on the areas of maximal correction each individual patient needs.

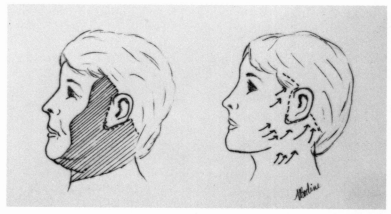

Fig. 7. Incisions for face-lift operation. Arrows show direction of "lift."

The skin is then dissected from the underlying facial tissue. Care is taken to leave several millimeters of fat on the under surface of the skin to protect its blood supply. This dissection is continued into the neck. The extent of this undermining is dictated by the degree of facial sagging of the patient.

After the facial skin is undermined, bleeding is controlled. At this point, some surgeons prefer to lift the underlying facial tissues, holding them in place with sutures in an effort to provide additional support for the sagging face. As there is no definite evidence that such plication helps produce a more satisfactory or lasting "lift," some surgeons omit this step.

The undermined skin of the face and neck is then pulled upward and backward and sutured into position in the temporal and mastoid regions, the points of maximum pull. Excess skin is removed as the skin is tailored to approximate the incision line. The surgeon makes sure that no significant tension or pull is exerted on the remaining areas of the incision line. Stress in areas other than the mastoid and temporal fixation points may cause stretching and widening of the scars in the postoperative period.

Some surgeons insert small rubber drains beneath the undermined skin to help drain collections of blood that may form in the early postoperative period.

After surgery is completed, a sterile dressing is applied, and the patient is transferred to a recovery area.

Postoperative Care

The average patient experiences little pain or discomfort following face-lift surgery. On the contrary, his face is usually numb because of injury to small nerve fibers that supply the skin. Regeneration of these fibers begins immediately and is usually complete in six to twelve weeks.

A sensation of pressure or tightness is common, but adjustment to it is rapid. Mild pain-relieving medications are given as necessary. If they don't relieve the discomfort, the surgeon is alerted to the possibility of an impending complication.

The patient is usually told to stay in bed and keep as quiet as possible to minimize the possibility of bleeding under the skin. A liquid diet is usually prescribed for forty-eight hours so that he does not have to use his large chewing muscles. Such activity could also cause postoperative bleeding.

The surgical dressing is usually removed forty-eight hours after the operation; and if rubber drains were placed beneath the skin, they are also removed at this time. Before these dressings are removed, the patient is warned that his face will appear swollen and locally discolored. The hair is usually in a state of disarray at this time and, although thorough shampooing is not permitted until the first sutures are removed, it can be carefully cleaned and unsnarled with a wet comb or dry shampoo.

The patient is usually discharged from the hospital after the dressing is removed. Gradual resumption of normal activities is recommended, and many patients can expect to return to work two weeks after the operation. Vigorous activity should be avoided for one month as it can temporarily elevate the blood pressure and result in hemorrhage under the facial skin. Some surgeons recommend use of facial slings at night for the first postoperative month in order to provide support for the healing tissue and to protect the face from inadvertent bumps that may occur while turning during sleep.

It is important to avoid direct exposure to the sun for several months after surgery as increased pigmentation and swelling of the facial skin may occur. Sun exposure, of course, accelerates deterioration and aging of the skin (see chapter 10).

The sutures in front of the ear are removed on the fifth postoperative day, and sutures in the temporal and mastoid hair on the seventh to tenth day. The sutures at the two points of maximal tension previously described are removed fourteen days after surgery.

Most women patients can enhance the results of the facelift with cosmetics. Many surgeons will arrange for their postoperative patients to learn techniques of cosmetic application. Cosmetics may be used after the sutures are removed on the fifth postoperative day. Frequent application of moisturizing cream is beneficial and many surgeons provide ointments to be applied to the incision.

Complications of the Face-Lift

Although serious complications occasionally occur after face-lift surgery, the convalescence of most patients is uneventful. The most common complication is bleeding beneath the undermined facial skin that results in formation of a localized collection of blood called a *hematoma*. This complication occurs in about 5 percent of face-lifts performed on women and in about 10 percent of male patients. The higher frequency of hematomas in males is probably related to the greater blood supply of their facial tissues.

Most hematomas are small and resolve spontaneously without consequence. Others are large enough to require evacuation in the surgeon's office. A small incision is made over the collection of blood, or the area is aspirated with a large needle. Occasionally a hematoma is large enough to require draining in the operating room. Because it is difficult to locally anesthetize the area that has already been operated upon, large hematomas are usually drained under general anesthesia in the operating room.

Although most hematomas form in the first few postoperative days, hemorrhage may occur later if the patient increases the blood pressure by lifting, straining, or some other vigorous exertion. Hematomas may also be precipitated by bumping the healing skin.

Excessive skin removal can cause other complications when it results in tightly sutured wounds that place excessive tension or strain on the undermined skin. Such stress can cause widening of the incision and an abnormally wide scar. However, such a scar can be revised at a later date, if it is objectionable.

Patches of hair may be lost from the temporal area as a consequence of excessive tension on the facial skin. Hair loss in this area may also occur if hair follicles are injured during the undermining process. While this is usually troublesome to women, it may be more of a problem to men. For this reason, when treating men patients some surgeons place the anterior portion of the incision at the edge of the temporal hairline.

The most devastating complication of face-lift surgery is localized skin injury that is secondary to impairment of blood supply caused by excessive tension or stress on the flap. Another cause of skin injury is the presence of a large hematoma that can affect the circulation by pressure from beneath. This complication is infrequent and in most cases only causes loss of the superficial layers of the skin (fig. 8). Patience and watchful waiting are in order when this happens, for in most cases a satisfactory result is obtained with spontaneous healing (figs. 9, 10, and 11). On occasion, however, measures such as skin grafting are required.

Fibers of small branches of the facial nerve, which control the movement of the muscles of facial expression, are occa-

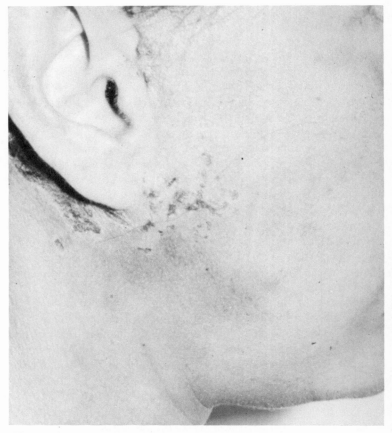

Fig. 8. Superficial skin loss following face-lift surgery.

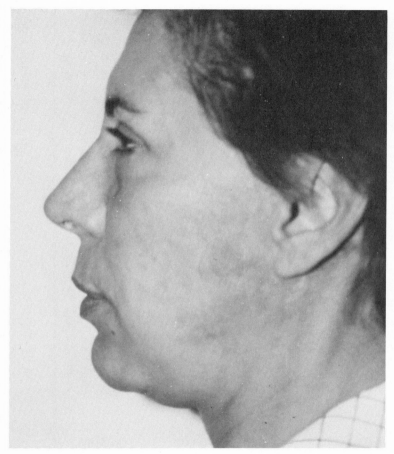

Fig. 9. Result after healing.

sionally injured during the face-lift. Such injury is usually temporary, with normal facial movement returning after regeneration of these nerve fibers.

Wound infection after the operation is extremely rare because of the excellent blood supply of the facial skin.

The Second Face-Lift

Many people ask how long it will be before recurrent

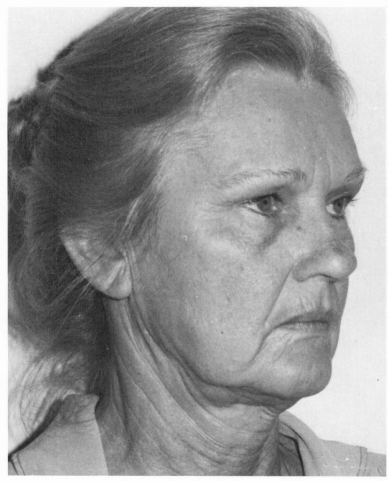

Fig. 10. Patient before face-lift.

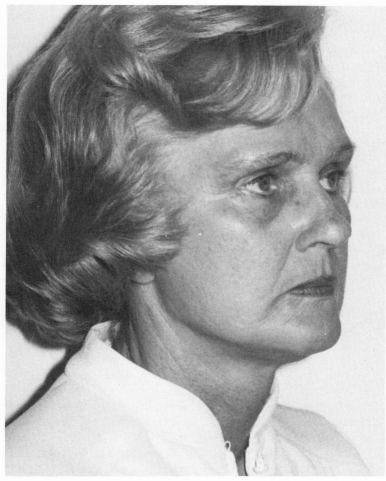

Fig. 11. After surgery has been performed.

sagging of the facial tissues necessitates a second face-lift. Although the average interval is five to ten years, in each case the interval depends on several factors. Perhaps the most important are the patient's age and skin condition at the time of the first operation. In general, the more advanced the facial sagging at the time of the first, the shorter the time will be before a second procedure is needed. In very advanced cases, recurrent sagging may occur as soon as one year after the operation. Thin, dry, brittle, weather-worn skin tends to behave in a similar fashion.

Patients whose weight fluctuates significantly after a face-lift are prone to an early recurrence of facial laxity. This happens because subcutaneous fat accumulates during periods of weight gain and stretches the facial skin, causing sagging as weight is lost.

Hereditary factors affecting the aging process also play an important role in how quickly the facial skin becomes lax again.

Modern Trends in Face-Lift Surgery

Because of the potential problems of excessive stress and tension if facial skin is stretched too tightly and the possibility of early recurrence of facial sagging regardless of the degree of stretch applied, some cosmetic facial surgeons now advocate a routine "mini-lift" or "tuck-up" procedure twelve to eighteen months after the initial face-lift. This is performed through the original incisions and consists of an abbreviated version of the initial operation. The tuck-up is generally performed as an office or outpatient procedure. The facial skin can usually be stretched more tightly at this time and it tolerates tension more predictably.

The trend in face-lift surgery is toward performance of the operation at an earlier age—frequently in the early forties when facial aging is at an early stage. The skin is healthier and more resilient, and the initial results are likely to last longer. Subsequent tuck-up procedures are generally more effective. One prominent cosmetic surgeon has termed this philosophy a program of "preventive maintenance."

Ancillary Procedures for the Aging Face

As previously stressed, certain characteristics of the aging face may not be significantly improved by the standard face-lift. Techniques used to alter such features are discussed in chapter 18.

The "Mini-Lift" Operation

Many patients who consult cosmetic facial surgeons inquire about the "mini-lift." Most cosmetic surgeons feel that this procedure is justified only in patients whose only manifestation of facial aging is laxity of skin in the cheek and jowls, without associated redundancy in the neck. This is an unusual condition.

The "mini-lift" is performed through an incision in the hairline of the temple that extends into the crease in front of the ear. The facial skin is undermined for a short distance and is then pulled back and the excess excised.

Most reputable cosmetic facial surgeons agree that the "mini-lift" produces relatively poor results that tend to last only a short time. Thus they advise most patients to consider a standard face-lift operation. As one prominent surgeon has stated, "a mini-lift gives a mini-result."

Special Considerations for Men

An increasing number of men are consulting cosmetic facial surgeons for face-lifts. The motivation of these men, while similar to that of women, may be slightly skewed toward economic and social factors.

When performed on a man, the face-lift operation differs in several ways. The surgeon may modify the incision so that scalp scars may not be as conspicuous, but the patient must understand that his hair style may require minor modification so it will conceal these scars. With the trend toward long hair, this is rarely a problem. As the facial skin is redistributed by the operation, the hair pattern is altered slightly. The sideburn is pulled closer to the ear. (A recent modification of the face-lift incision preserves the normal sideburn position.) The skin of the upper neck, which is ultimately placed behind the ear, continues to grow and thus this area usually requires postoperative shaving.

Hematomas are more common after a male face-lift as the skin is thicker and it contains a more extensive network of blood vessels. If the operation is complicated by hair loss in the temple, the affected area may be more difficult to camouflage. Hair transplantation (see chapter 22) may be required if this area cannot be covered by adjacent hair. Such measures, however, are unusual.

12

Blepharoplasty— Cosmetic Surgery of the Eyelids

Blepharoplasty is an operation designed to correct abnormalities in the appearance of the eyelids occurring as a result of aging or various hereditary factors (*blepharo*—eyelid; *plasty*—repair). The eyes are the most expressive features of the human face, largely because of subtle variations in the eyelids that result from activity of the underlying muscles (see chapter 9). But a price must be paid for such animation, and this price is extracted in the form of the wrinkling and sagging of skin that is a hallmark of aging.

The eyelids are among the first areas of the face to exhibit signs of aging. This begins with development of "laugh lines" or "crow's-feet" at the outer corners of the eyes during the late twenties or early thirties (fig. 1). Next, sagging of the skin of the upper lid begins and produces hooding of the lid that is especially marked in its outer half (fig. 2). Fat that lies in compartments between the skin and muscle of the lower lids may protrude, producing pouches or "bags" that result in a "tired" or "sad" look (fig. 3). Sagging of the outer corner of the eyelid and eyebrows reinforces this impression (fig. 4).

Although most blepharoplasties are performed to alleviate these manifestations of aging, this procedure is sometimes valuable to younger patients. Some people exhibit eyelid puf-

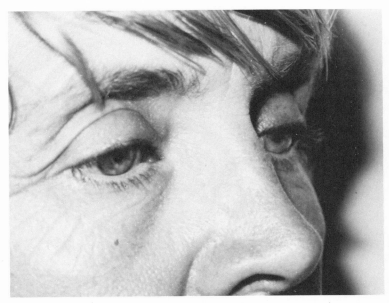

Fig. 1. "Crow's-feet" at the outer corner of the eyes.

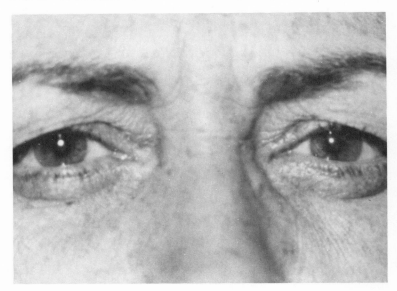

Fig. 2. "Hooding" of the upper eyelid, most marked on the outside.

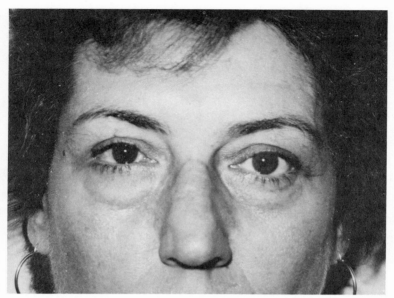

Fig. 3. Fat protrusion producing "bags" beneath the lower eyelids.

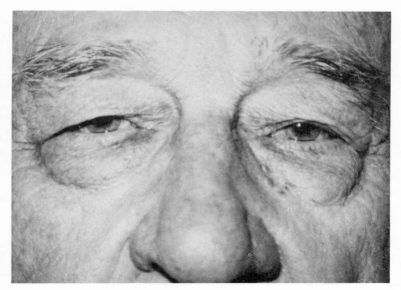

Fig. 4. Sagging of the outer corner of the eye.

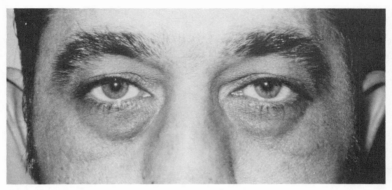

Fig. 5. Eyelid puffiness in a young adult.

finess, particularly in the lower lids, at an early age (fig. 5). This deformity—thought to be hereditary—is caused by protrusion of fat through the weakened membrane (*orbital septum*) that normally confines this tissue to its compartments around the eye.

The blepharoplasty consists of removal of excess skin, muscle, and fat from around the eyelid. Because the eyes are the focal point of the face, this is one of the most commonly requested cosmetic facial procedures, and a successful blepharoplasty is one of the most satisfying of all cosmetic procedures for both patient and surgeon. This operation is frequently performed in conjunction with the face-lift, but it is often performed alone, as eyelid sagging generally occurs five to ten years before significant relaxation of the facial skin.

The History of Blepharoplasty

Study and classification of eyelid abnormalities that occur secondary to aging, or as a result of hereditary factors, began in the mid-nineteenth century. Although surgical correction of these deformities was not performed for cosmetic reasons, some physicians recognized that redundant eyelid skin overhanging the visual fields of the eye caused visual abnormalities, and surgical procedures were devised to correct them. An improvement in appearance after these operations was noted, but was considered an incidental benefit.

With the gradual acceptance of cosmetic facial surgery by the medical profession and the public, techniques of blepharoplasty have evolved to the point that this procedure—when patients are properly selected—is a reliable approach to the rejuvenation of sagging, puffy eyelids.

Anatomy of the Eyelids

The eyelids are delicate structures that protect the eyes from irritation and injury. They also serve as a pump mechanism that aids in draining tears. The skeleton of the eyelids, the *tarsus* or *tarsal plate* is a rigid structure comprised of dense fibrous tissue that has a cartilagelike consistency.

A thin membrane—*the orbital septum*—extends from the edges of the tarsal plates to attach to the orbital margins of the bony facial skeleton. Behind this septum are compartments containing fat tissue that cushion the eyeball. There are two or three separate compartments in each lid. Weakening of the orbital septum as a result of aging or hereditary factors may allow this fat to protrude, applying pressure to the overlying skin and resulting in pouches or "bags" around the eye.

The eyelid skin is thin and delicate. A characteristic furrow, the *superior palpebral fold* (fig. 6) is present in the upper

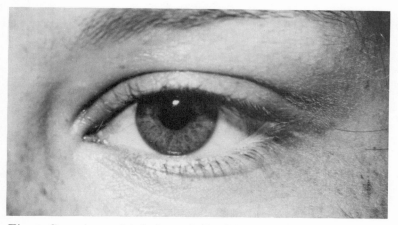

Fig. 6. Superior and inferior palpebral folds of eyelids.

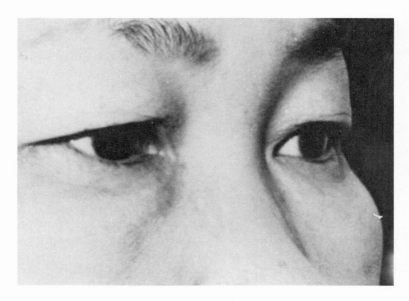

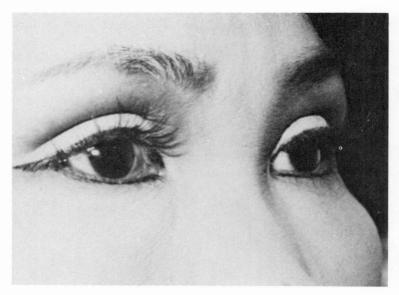

Fig. 7. Creation of a "double eyelid" in the Oriental eye,
(a) preoperative, (b) postoperative.

lid when the eye is open. This fold, which marks the edge of the tarsal plate, is absent in approximately 50 percent of Orientals (figs. 7*a* and *b*). It is a characteristic determined by hereditary factors. Creation of an "upper lid fold" is a commonly performed cosmetic procedure in the Orient and in other areas that have a large Oriental population. This operation is a modification of the basic blepharoplasty procedure.

The lower lid exhibits a similar furrow, the *inferior palpebral fold* (fig. 6), but this crease is frequently absent and usually disappears in childhood.

A third crease is often noted where the lower eyelid skin joins the cheek. This line of demarcation often becomes more apparent with increasing age. It marks the lower extent of puffiness in association with swelling or "bags" of the lid.

Numerous hairs or eyelashes project from the margins of each lid. These lashes show marked individual variation in thickness, length, and number and are generally longer and thicker in the upper lids.

Beneath the eyelid skin is the *orbicularis oculi* muscle, which surrounds the eye in a circular fashion and is responsible for closing the eyelids as well as aiding the flow of tears. Contraction of this muscle causes the "crow's-feet" at the outer edge of the eye. The upper lid is opened by contraction of a small muscle (*levator palpebrae superioris*) that attaches to the tarsal plate and skin of the upper lid. The attachments of this muscle to the skin at the edge of the tarsus produce the superior palpebral fold.

Characteristics of the Youthful and Aging Eye

Although there is significant individual variation in the configuration of the youthful eye, certain characteristics are common. The outer edge of the eye is generally higher than the inner border. This characteristic, of course, is more dramatic in the Oriental, but is noted to some degree in the white and black races. During aging, the outer edge tends to sag while the inner edge remains stationary.

The youthful eye seems wide and large when the lids are

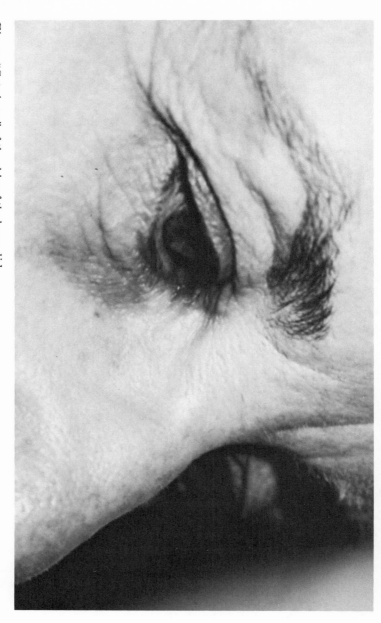

Fig. 8. "Crêpiness" of the skin of the lower lid.

open, giving an impression of alertness. Due to sagging of eyelid skin and protrusion of fat, the aging eye appears less wide, adding to the illusion of fatigue or sadness.

Both lids are relatively wrinkle-free during youth, but as we have seen, characteristic patterns of wrinkling develop during aging.

The youthful brow characteristically forms an arch, with its highest point near the junction of the outer and middle thirds of the eye. With increasing age, the brow begins to droop, and the distance between the brow and the upper eyelid margin decreases. Some women disguise this sagging by plucking the eyebrows and creating an arching brow with a brow pencil.

Eyelid Deformities That Can Be Corrected by Blepharoplasty

Several types of eyelid deformities can be corrected by the blepharoplasty operation. Perhaps the most common is wrinkling and sagging of redundant eyelid skin. Sagging obscures the upper lid fold and frequently causes a hoodlike deformity of the upper lid, particularly on the outside. Wrinkling of the skin of the lower lid produces a crepey, tissue paper appearance that detracts from the youthful vitality of the lid (fig. 8).

The second most common deformity is produced by the herniation of periorbital fat previously described. This protrusion is usually more noticeable near the inner corners of the lids and causes a puffy appearance sometimes referred to as "pouches" or "bags." Fat protrusion is often associated with the skin wrinkling and redundancy of aging but sometimes occurs at an earlier age as a consequence of heredity. This deformity produces a tired or sad appearance and often suggests that a person overindulges in alcohol or suffers from insomnia.

A third condition that can be aided by blepharoplasty is the presence of a bulge just below the edge of the lower lid (fig. 9). This bulge, which becomes more prominent when smiling, develops as a result of overuse of the orbicularis oculi muscle—frequently because of squinting in strong sunlight.

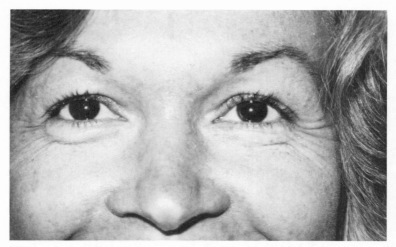

Fig. 9. Bulge under lower lid produced by contraction of the orbicularis oculi muscle.

People with highly animated faces are also likely to develop this bulge.

Baggy Eyelids as a Symptom

Correction of baggy eyelids is often sought for other than cosmetic reasons. Many people with redundancy of the upper lid skin complain of a sensation of heaviness. Fatigue of the upper eyelid muscles can occur as a result of the constant strain of opening the heavy lid—a factor that may contribute to the "tired" look of people with this condition. Hooding of the upper lid skin may also interfere with vision by obstructing the upper-outer visual field.

Puffiness of the lower lid produces an appearance of chronic fatigue that can suggest overwork, insomnia, or even overindulgence in alcohol. Such impressions can have subtle social and economic effects, and this is one reason that an increasing number of men are requesting blepharoplasty.

What a Blepharoplasty Will Not Do

The candidate for cosmetic eyelid surgery should be aware

that some eyelid deformities cannot be completely corrected by blepharoplasty. This operation rarely results in complete eradication of every wrinkle in the lower lid producing the smooth skin of youth. People with animated faces must realize that wrinkles that occur when they smile or show other forms of expression will not be eliminated—although they may be improved—by blepharoplasty. The "crow's-feet" at the outer edge of the eyes often show little change after a successful operation.

Large "bags" of the lower lids may not be totally removed by the blepharoplasty, and redundancy of the upper lid skin related to sagging of the eyebrow is not completely relieved either. Ancillary procedures designed to improve these defects in conjunction with blepharoplasty are discussed in a following section.

Selecting Candidates
for Blepharoplasty

Candidates for blepharoplasty are carefully evaluated by the cosmetic facial surgeon. It is particularly important that the presence of any medical disorders that may contribute to the development of baggy eyelids be excluded before surgery. These include disorders of the thyroid gland, kidneys, and cardiovascular system. The presence of such problems can usually be detected during the interview and physical examination, but occasionally laboratory tests are required. Eyelid puffiness may be improved after these conditions are controlled but if it persists, blepharoplasty may be safely performed in most cases.

The surgeon is also concerned with the presence of symptoms that indicate disorders of the eyes themselves. Such symptoms include visual blurring, double vision, excessive tearing or dryness of the eyes, and chronic irritation of the eyelids. Sharpness of vision is carefully documented. Many cosmetic facial surgeons insist on a formal consultation with an ophthalmologist prior to blepharoplasty in order to be sure to exclude pre-existing abnormalities of the eye.

It is also important to assess the general nature of the eyelid skin. Thickened eyelid skin tends to remain bruised and swollen longer than thin skin, and maturation of the scar may take longer. In older people, the eyelid margin may be overly relaxed, exhibiting a tendency to pull away from the eye. In many cases, the operation must be modified to insure that the lower lid is not permanently drawn away from the eye.

Gentle pressure on the lids while closed helps the surgeon determine how much protruding fat contributes to the eyelid deformity. Pressure results in bulging of fat beneath the skin when the orbital septum is weakened.

The presence of a sagging eyebrow, large lower lid "bags," and other conditions previously discussed that are not correctable by blepharoplasty alone are noted during the examination.

The emotional makeup of the prospective patient—including motivational factors and expectations—is carefully evaluated. It is important that the patient's expectations be realistic, and that it is understood that the goal of blepharoplasty is improvement in the appearance of the eyelids and not absolute perfection. Occasionally a patient may be asked to undergo psychological or psychiatric evaluation prior to acceptance for surgery if the surgeon does not feel comfortable with the patient's motives for surgery or his general emotional makeup.

Preparation for Blepharoplasty

The prospective patient is carefully counselled about important details of the operation and postoperative period. The location and extent of scars are carefully discussed, and the process of scar maturation is described. Possible complications of the operation are explained and the patient is encouraged to ask questions about points he does not fully understand. Literature about important things discussed in the preoperative interview may be provided so that the patient is further able to review these matters.

Photographs of the eyes are taken and carefully reviewed with the patient. The areas to be corrected are identified, and associated defects and asymmetries which the patient may not be aware of are pointed out.

The goals and limitations of the operation are then reviewed before executing an informed consent agreement that gives the surgeon permission to operate. The final discussion of the limitations of the procedure is of particular importance for patients who exhibit eyelid deformities that are not correctable by blepharoplasty alone. As is the case with most cosmetic operations, blepharoplasty has been glamorized and sensationalized to the point that there are often misconceptions about the results of surgery.

Fees for blepharoplasty are usually paid in advance, and a member of the surgeon's office staff generally discusses this matter with the patient before final scheduling of surgery (see chapter 1).

The patient is instructed to avoid the use of aspirin as it may interfere with the clotting mechanism of the blood, resulting in increased operative or postoperative bleeding. Instructions are also given regarding the use of other medications the patient may be taking.

Hospital vs. Office Surgery

If the blepharoplasty is to be performed in a hospital operating room, the patient is usually admitted on the evening before surgery to undergo preoperative physical examinations and laboratory tests. An increasing number of blepharoplasties, however, are being performed in outpatient surgical facilities, including office operating rooms or ambulatory care units. Patients undergoing operations in facilities of this type usually have their physical examination and laboratory tests on the day before surgery and arrive at the operating area several hours before surgery. Such patients are instructed to avoid food for six to eight hours before the operation to minimize the chance of vomiting.

Preoperative Medication

Sedative medication may be given by mouth several hours

before surgery and reinforced with injections one hour before.

Anesthesia for Blepharoplasty

Blepharoplasty is most frequently performed under local anesthesia (see chapter 6), although some surgeons use general anesthesia. If local anesthesia is chosen, the solution is infiltrated beneath the eyelid skin with a small hypodermic needle. If surgery is to be performed under general anesthesia, an anesthesiologist will be present to administer the anesthetic.

The Blepharoplasty Operation

The facial skin is cleaned with an antiseptic solution and sterile drapes are placed around the operative field to prevent contamination.

The incision lines are carefully marked before the anesthetic solution is infiltrated. Many surgeons prefer to do this marking with the patient sitting up. The upper and lower lid incisions generally are like those shown in figure 10 but may vary somewhat depending on the extent and location of redundant skin. Both incisions generally extend into the "crow's-feet" at the external edge of the eye and after maturation are scarcely perceptible.

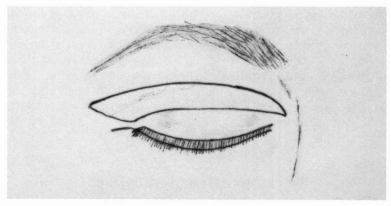

Fig. 10. Incisions for blepharoplasty.

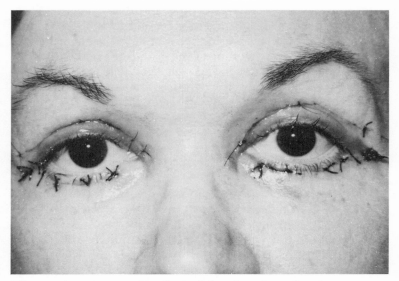

Fig. 11. Appearance after the incisions have been closed.

The upper lid blepharoplasty is usually performed first. Redundant skin of the lid is excised and a strip of underlying orbicularis oculi muscle is removed. If fat is to be removed, the orbital septum is then incised and the appropriate amount of fat excised. The skin is then closed with sutures (fig. 11).

Next, the skin of the lower lid is incised and elevated from its underlying attachments (undermined) to the level of the lower bony margin of the orbit. In some patients, the skin and underlying orbicularis oculi muscle is elevated as a unit, while in others the skin is separated from the muscle. If necessary, fat is removed after incision of the orbital septum. The undermined lower lid skin is then stretched upward and excess skin carefully removed. Finally, the incision is closed with sutures.

Postoperative Care

Immediately after the procedure is completed, light dressings are placed over the eyes, care being taken to avoid pressure. Iced compresses are then placed over the dressing to minimize postoperative swelling and discoloration. These iced compresses are continued for twenty-four hours.

The patient is placed at his bed rest with the head elevated to further minimize swelling of the eyelids. Periodically, ointment is placed in his eyes and over the incision lines to protect the eye and minimize crusting of the suture line.

There is usually little pain or discomfort after the blepharoplasty. Indeed, severe eye pain suggests the possibility of a complication and necessitates careful inspection of the eye. Most patients notice a definite sensation of tightness, especially in the lower lids. This sensation frequently persists for several weeks.

If the operation was performed in a hospital, the patient is usually discharged on the morning after surgery with instructions to continue applying iced compresses for twenty-four hours after surgery. Ointment is applied to the suture lines three or four times a day and placed in the eye at night. If the eyes are dry, artificial tears are used as often as necessary.

At the time of discharge, the eyelids are frequently swollen and discolored. Much of this discoloration disappears in seven to ten days, but the rate of resolution in an individual varies. Many patients wear sunglasses during this period and most are able to resume their normal activities several days after surgery.

The sutures are removed on the third postoperative day. Frequently, several stitches at the outer aspect of the lids are left in place until the fifth day. This is the point of maximal tension on the suture line, and earlier removal could possibly predispose to separation of the skin edges.

Use of cosmetics to camouflage residual discoloration can begin after all the sutures are removed. The skin can also be carefully cleansed with soap and water at this time. Some surgeons recommend massage of the outer incisions with lanolin or other substances to hasten maturation of the scar.

Although most eyelid swelling is resolved in two to three weeks, complete resolution may require three to four months. Consequently, the result of the operation cannot be finally appraised until this time. (Figures 12, 13, 14, 15, 17, and 18 show before and after pictures of patients.)

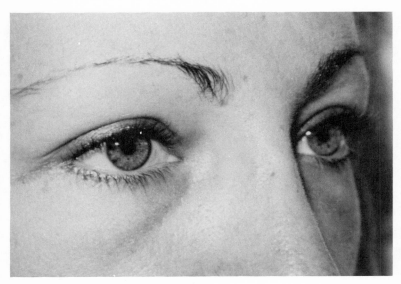

Fig. 12. Before the blepharoplasty.

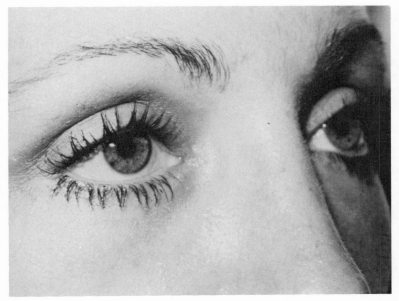

Fig. 13. The same person after surgery.

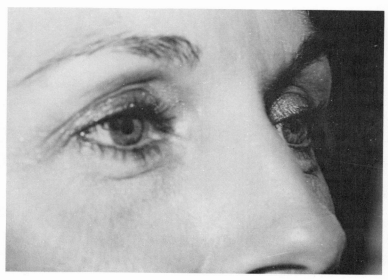

Fig. 14. Another patient prior to surgery.

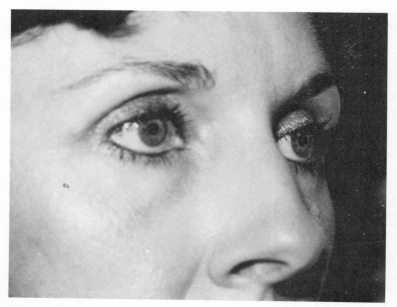

Fig. 15. The results of the operation.

Complications of Blepharoplasty

Although the postoperative course in most patients undergoing blepharoplasty is uneventful, as in any surgical procedure, complications can occur.

Postoperative bleeding is unusual but it may necessitate return to the operating room. Localized collections of blood beneath the undermined skin (hematoma) occasionally occur and may require draining.

Perhaps the most common complication of this operation is development of small white pustules called *milia* along the incision line, most often in the upper lid (fig. 16). The milia are caused by growth of skin along the suture. This skin becomes trapped beneath the lid surface and forms small cysts. Milia are easily removed in the surgeon's office without anesthesia and thus are essentially inconsequential. The upper lid suture is removed on the second postoperative day in an effort to prevent formation of milia.

Dryness of the eyes may be a temporary aftereffect of blepharoplasty. Artificial tear preparations are prescribed until normal tearing returns. Occasionally a patient complains of excessive tearing. This may be secondary to minor irritation or in some cases to malfunction of the tear pump mechanism of the lower lid muscle described previously. In most cases, excessive tearing is only temporary.

Wound infection is extremely rare because of the excellent blood supply of the eyelids. For similar reasons, the incisions heal rapidly and scars are nearly imperceptible after maturation. Occasionally the outer aspect of the upper or lower lid incisions separates after suture removal. If this occurs, temporary replacement of the stitch results in excellent healing.

Sometimes a patient develops prolonged swelling and discoloration of the eyelids. The reasons for this are not known, but they may be related to obscure individual healing factors.

Excessive skin removal during blepharoplasty can result in several complications. In the upper lid, this may cause inability to close the eye (*lagophthalmos*). The amount of skin excision in the upper lid is planned so that after closure of the wound the eyes do not close completely. By the morning after surgery, however, complete closure should be possible.

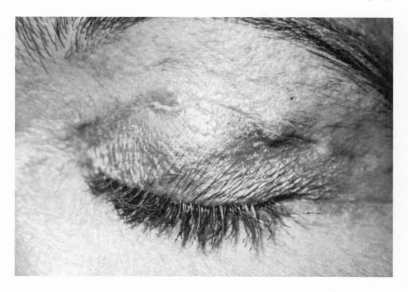

Fig. 16. Milia along upper eyelid incision.

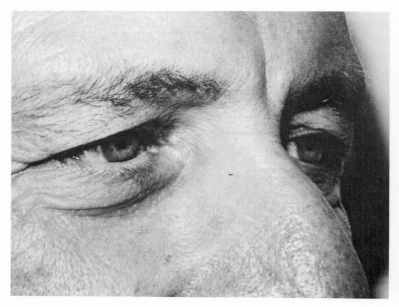

Fig. 17. Preoperative appearance.

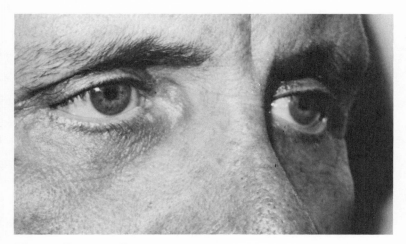

Fig. 18. Postoperative appearance.

Excessive removal of lower lid skin may pull the lid margin down resulting in an *ectropion*. This problem is difficult to correct, and for this reason cosmetic facial surgeons are conservative when performing lower lid blepharoplasty. It is better to have several residual wrinkles in the lower lid than to have ectropion result from attempts to maximally tighten the lower lid skin.

The most devastating complication of blepharoplasty is visual impairment or blindness. This is extremely rare and has been reported in only a handful of patients. The reason blindness occurs remains uncertain. Most surgeons, however, feel that postoperative bleeding into the structures around the eye is responsible. Such hemorrhage causes an increase in pressure around the eye that may interfere with blood flow to the visual areas. Bleeding into this area is initially marked by pain and protrusion of the eye. These warning signs necessitate prompt evaluation and may require exploration of the operative site to find the bleeding point.

Temporary blurring of vision may last for several days after blepharoplasty as a result of the irritation and swelling of the eye. It may be minimized by keeping the eye moist with artificial tears. Occasionally other types of eye drops may be necessary.

Ancillary Procedures for the Aging Eye

There are supplementary procedures available to correct signs of aging that are not amenable to blepharoplasty alone. Perhaps the most commonly performed ancillary procedure is the "brow lift," which is designed to elevate the sagging eyebrow and restore its youthful sweep. This operation can be performed using an incision directly over the eyebrow or can be done in conjunction with the face-lift procedure through the incisions used for that operation (see chapter 11).

The large bags that may be present at the junction of the lower eyelid and cheek skin may require direct excision if they are not significantly improved by blepharoplasty. The scars from this procedure are usually well camouflaged after maturation.

Residual fine wrinkling of skin of the lower lid can often be improved by a chemical peel of the lids (see chapter 19). This procedure is usually performed several months after the blepharoplasty.

13

Correcting the Sagging Eyebrow

The youthful eyebrow sweeps across the area above the upper eyelid in the form of an arched bow. It is somewhat higher at its outer edge (fig. 1). Sagging of the brow is a common accompaniment of facial aging. This drooping tends to be most marked in the outer half of the brow. It is a major factor in creating the hooded appearance of the upper lid that tends to obscure the edge of the eyelid and produces a sad or tired look (fig 2). As discussed in chapter 12, redundancy of the upper eyelid skin is the other factor contributing to this hooding effect.

For many patients who want facial rejuvenation, elevation of the brow may be the key to restoring a youthful appearance, as it makes the difference between a satisfactory postoperative result and a truly outstanding result. Blepharoplasty alone cannot eliminate the effects of a drooping brow and in many cases actually tends to accentuate this sagging as the brow is pulled closer to the upper lid when eyelid skin is removed.

The Structure and Function of the Eyebrow

The eyebrow is formed by multiple hairs that project from

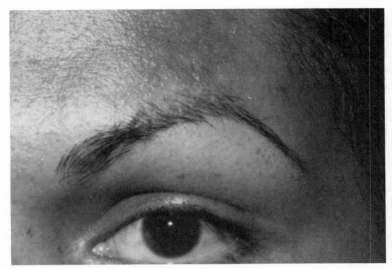

Fig. 1. The youthful eyebrow resembles an arched bow. The highest point of this arch is located between the outer edge of the lids and pupil.

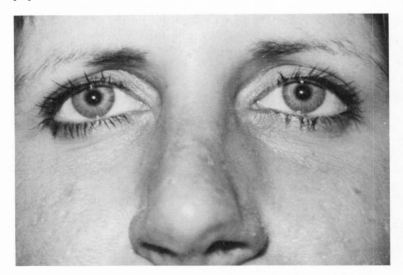

Fig. 2. Drooping of the eyebrow is generally most marked in the outer half. Sagging produces a hood over the aspect of the upper lid resulting in a sad or tired look.

the skin at the junction of the forehead and eyelid. A definite bony ridge can easily be felt beneath the brow. The hairs of the brow vary greatly in length, thickness, and number, tending to be thicker and more numerous in men. The hair of the brow frequently does not grow back if it is removed. Many women take advantage of this by plucking the eyebrows and using eyebrow pencil to create an artificial brow with the higher, more delicate arch characteristic of youth.

The normal brow lies ten to twelve millimeters above the edge of the upper eyelid and the highest point of its arch is between the outer edge of the eyelids and the pupil. The height and shape of the brow varies among individuals, but men's brows tend to be somewhat lower.

The skin of the eyebrow is thicker than the delicate eyelid skin. Beneath this skin lie several muscles that serve to move the brow (see chapter 9). Contraction of the orbicularis occuli muscle depresses the brow while the frontalis muscle elevates it. Contraction of the corrugator supercilii muscles pulls the brows inward and is responsible for the vertical "frown lines" that are characteristic of aging. The subtle variations in position of the brow allowed by selective activity of these muscles make them important to facial expression.

The function of the eyebrows is to assist the lids in protecting the eye. In response to irritants and other noxious substances, the lids close and the eyebrows contract, producing a squint. In an urban environment, perhaps the most frequent cause of squinting is exposure to bright sunlight. As described in chapter 9, excessive use of the facial muscles produces wrinkles. Squinting contributes to formation of the vertical frown lines as well as the "crow's-feet" radiating from the outside corner of the eye.

Surgical Elevation of the Eyebrow

Several surgical procedures have been advocated for restoring the vibrant, youthful appearance of the eyebrow. These procedures, called "brow lifts," offer other advantages besides the obvious improvement in the position and shape of the brow. Most brow lift procedures eliminate or improve the "crow's-feet" at the outside corner of the eye. This procedure, in the presence of a sagging brow, enhances the results of an upper lid blepharoplasty. The blepharoplasty may actually increase such sagging in some patients because excessive skin excision pulls the brow closer to the eyelid margin.

The locations of incisions for different brow lift procedures are diagrammed in figure 3. A general principle of brow lift surgery is that the degree of brow elevation increases as the incision approaches the brow. Thus the operation utilizing an incision directly over the brow produces a greater brow lift than incisions in the hairline. Unfortunately, the resulting scar is more noticeable as the incision approaches the brow.

Although the sagging eyebrow is not corrected by the standard face-lift operation, slight degrees of brow depression can frequently be corrected during the operation by extending dissection into the temple. The possibility of injury to the branch of the facial nerve that moves the forehead and eye muscles is slightly increased by this procedure, but the

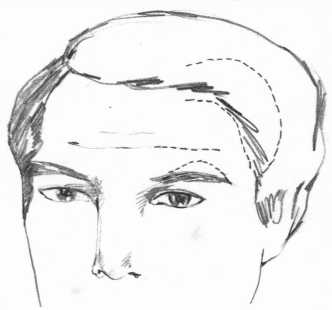

Fig. 3. Location of various incisions used for elevating the sagging eyebrow.

surgeon is aware of the location of this nerve and makes every effort to avoid injury.

Incisions in the hairline of the temporal area may also satisfactorily correct a mild sagging of the brow. Marked sagging, however, can be satisfactorily corrected by an incision directly over the brow. If the resulting scar is visible, it can be satisfactorily covered with eyebrow pencil or other cosmetics. As the scar cannot be covered in this manner by the few men who would benefit from a brow lift, some surgeons recommend placing the incision in a horizontal wrinkle line just above the brow. As the resulting scar will fall in a natural wrinkle line, it will be camouflaged after maturation.

A method of removing sagging skin beneath the eyebrow using an incision directly below the edge of the brow has also been described. This operation, of course, will not elevate the brow itself.

Some surgeons suggest that the results of the brow lift are enhanced by excision of the nerves or muscles that move the brow. The penalty for this excision, of course, is the lessening of brow animation.

Selection of Patients for the Brow Lift

Any patient with sagging eyebrows is a potential candidate for the brow lift operation. Most patients who request cosmetic surgery for rejuvenation of the aging eye are not aware of the contribution of the eyebrow to their appearance. Consequently, the surgeon must frequently point out and explain the significance of this problem and the benefits that may be expected from its correction.

In assessing the contribution of a sagging brow to the aging eye, the surgeon first determines the position of the brow in relation to the bony *supraorbital ridge*. If the brow is at, or above, this level, sagging is generally not significant. Excessive redundancy and hooding of the skin of the outer aspect of the upper eyelids is frequently caused by drooping of the outer part of the brow. It requires a brow lift in conjunction with blepharoplasty for optimal correction. Elevation of the brow with the finger (fig. 4) will show the expected

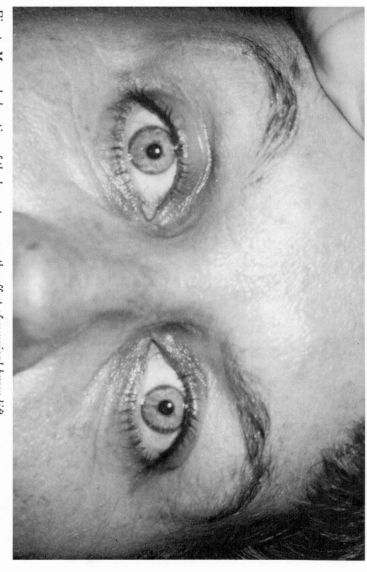

Fig. 4. Manual elevation of the brow to assess the effect of surgical brow lift.

benefit of surgery, although the final degree of elevation may not be exactly the same.

The remainder of the interview and examination is directed toward evaluating other features of the eye as described in the section on blepharoplasty (see chapter 12). Psychological factors (i.e., motives and expectations) as well as the importance of the general health of the patient are assessed as discussed in previous chapters.

The patient is then counselled about important details of the surgical procedure and postoperative period. Particular emphasis is placed on the location and extent of scars that may result from the brow lift and the ways in which they can be camouflaged. This is of particular importance to men, who cannot hide scars with makeup. Possible complications are discussed, and the patient is encouraged to ask questions about things he does not completely understand. An informed consent agreement giving the surgeon permission to perform the operation is prepared.

As brow lift surgery is almost always performed in conjunction with blepharoplasty, final preoperative instructions are similar to those covered in chapter 12. If the patient has plucked the brows and recreated them with eyebrow pencil, it is important that they be penciled at the proper location on arrival in the operating room so that the surgeon can mark his incision in the proper place.

As the blepharoplasty, the brow lift operation may be performed either in a hospital operating room or an outpatient surgical facility. Preoperative sedatives are administered, and upon arrival in the operating room an intravenous infusion is started through which additional medication can be given if necessary.

Anesthesia for the Brow Lift

Although most brow lift procedures are performed under local anesthesia, some surgeons perform this operation under general anesthesia (see chapter 6).

The Brow Lift Operation

The brow lift is usually performed before the upper lid blepharoplasty because elevation of the brow lessens hooding of the eyelid skin and decreases the amount of skin that must be excised from the lid.

With the patient sitting up, the skin incisions are marked. The size and configuration of these incisions varies depending on the extent to which the brow must be elevated and the type of brow lift to be performed. Typical incisions for brow lift operations, made just above the eyebrow, in a forehead crease above the brow, and in the hairline, are shown in figure 5.

After the anesthetic solution is injected, the skin is excised and undermined. Subcutaneous sutures of nylon or other material that will remain in the wound permanently are used to suspend the brow. If such sutures are not used, premature sagging of the brow may occur. The skin edges are closed and ointment or a dressing is applied to the wound.

Postoperative Care

Pain or discomfort is usually minimal after the brow lift operation. Swelling and discoloration of the eyes occurs in all patients but has generally faded in seven to ten days. Iced compresses are applied to the eyes for twenty-four hours after surgery in order to minimize swelling and discoloration.

If a gauze dressing was applied to the brow, it is removed on the first day after surgery. The patient is told to apply ointment to the wound several times a day to prevent crusting over the incision.

Skin stitches are removed on the third or fourth postoperative day and the healing wound is stabilized with skin tapes for the following week. After removal of this tape, cosmetics and eyebrow pencil can be applied to camouflage the scar.

The scar initially has a reddish appearance but over the ensuing six to twelve months matures into a thin, white line that is easily covered with makeup.

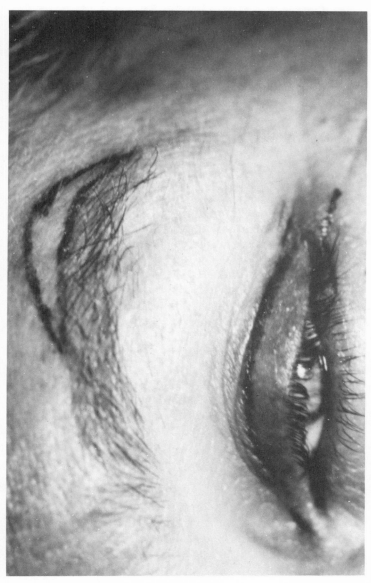

Fig. 5. Typical skin excision for suprabrow lift.

Complications of the Brow Lift

Complications following brow lift surgery are unusual and are related to the type of operation performed. When the incision is placed in the hairline there is apt to be a higher incidence of complications as more extensive undermining of the forehead skin is needed to adequately elevate the brow. These procedures may be complicated by postoperative bleeding under the skin, forming a hematoma that may require incision and drainage.

Injury to the small branches of the facial nerve that move the muscles of the forehead and eye can occur, and damage to small nerve fibers responsible for sensations of pain and touch in these areas occasionally occurs. Although such nerve injuries frequently heal, damage may be permanent.

The major complication of operations performed directly over the brow is a noticeable scar. Such scars are particularly troublesome to men, who are not accustomed to covering facial blemishes with makeup. Most scars improve significantly during maturation, but unsightly scars still present a year after surgery may benefit from revision (see chapter 7).

Infection is seldom a problem after the eyebrow lift, but it may occur after any of the various surgical procedures. If a brow lift is complicated by infection, a more visible scar may result.

At times the degree of correction from brow lift surgery may not be optimal. As previously noted, adequate, lasting correction of the sagging brow is easiest to obtain when the incision is close to the brow (figs. 6 and 7). Occasionally the brow is overcorrected, producing an undesirable "startled" or "surprised" look. In some cases, correction may be asymmetrical. Meticulous attention to detail during the operation minimizes the chance of these problems, but in spite of the efforts of the surgeon such complications can be caused by factors beyond his control. Hair loss is an infrequent complication of brow lift operations, but it occasionally occurs after any of the available surgical procedures.

The brow lift operation is a valuable adjunct to treatment of the aging face. In most cases the advantages of this opera-

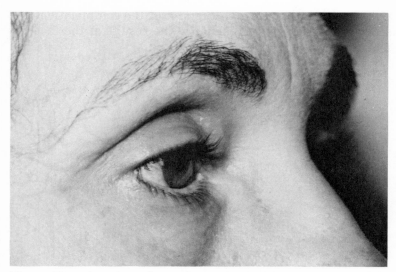

Fig. 6. Elevation of sagging eyebrow with incision in upper margin of brow (suprabrow lift), preoperative view.

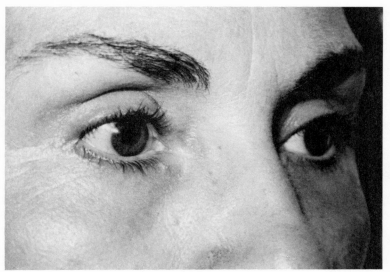

Fig. 7. Postoperative view of patient.

tion significantly outweigh the risk of the complications described and they greatly enhance the results of the face-lift and blepharoplasty procedures.

14

Cosmetic Surgery of the Nose

As the nose is the most prominent feature of the face, its size and shape are of major importance in facial appearance. Many people are dissatisfied with the configuration of their noses, and so *rhinoplasty*—an operation designed to modify the nasal appearance—is now the most commonly performed cosmetic facial operation. Rhinoplasty is frequently done in conjunction with surgical manipulation of the nasal septum (the partition of bone and cartilage that divides the inside of the nose into two separate cavities), and this combined operation is called *septorhinoplasty*.

History of Rhinoplasty

Operations to correct nasal deformities that resulted from injury were described by Egyptian surgeons before 1600 B.C. Sophisticated procedures for nasal reconstruction were devised by surgeons of ancient India and were revived by Italian surgeons during the Middle Ages. Cosmetic surgery of the nose, however, is relatively new. It was born in the late nineteenth century. Although there is some controversy about who was the first surgeon to perform cosmetic nasal surgery using incisions inside the nose, a German orthopedic surgeon,

Dr. Jacques Joseph, is considered the father of modern rhino-plasty. Dr. Joseph jealously guarded his techniques, and it was not until the early twentieth century that he agreed to teach his method to other surgeons. Although many technical refinements have been devised since then, the basic surgical method of rhinoplasty remains essentially unchanged.

Rhinoplasty is most frequently performed during early adulthood, but an increasing number of middle-aged people are requesting it. Cosmetic nasal surgery is also performed to reverse the effects of aging on the nose.

Anatomy of the Nose

The most important determinant of nasal shape is the configuration of the framework or skeleton, formed by bone and cartilage. The rigid upper half of the nose is formed by two paired nasal bones that are attached to a firm buttress of bone projecting from the *frontal bone* above and to two small projections from the *maxillary bone* on each side (fig. 1).

The lower, relatively mobile half of the nasal skeleton is formed by cartilage. The framework of the tip consists of paired cartilages (the lower lateral or *alar* cartilages), which are arranged in archlike fashion around the nostrils. The paired upper lateral cartilages bridge the gap between the nasal bones and *alar* cartilages, completing the cartilaginous skeleton (fig. 2).

The nasal skin is of varying thickness in different areas of the nose. Over the tip and lower third of the nose, the skin and underlying (subcutaneous) tissue is relatively thick and well-endowed with glands that produce sebaceous material. Irritation of the skin in this area may result in an increased thickness that in extreme cases produces a grotesque deformity known as *rhinophyma*. The skin and subcutaneous tissue gradually thins over the upper cartilaginous framework and is thinnest at the junction of the cartilaginous and bony skeletons. The nasal skin then increases in thickness over the bony skeleton. It is relatively thick at the junction of the nose and forehead (nasal root). The thickness and consistency of nasal skin, of course, exhibits considerable individual, sexual, and racial differences.

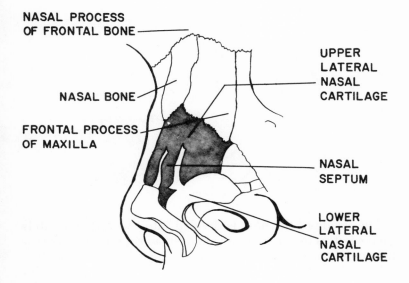

Fig. 1. The nasal skeleton. Note the horseshoe or arched configuration of the lower lateral (alar) cartilages.

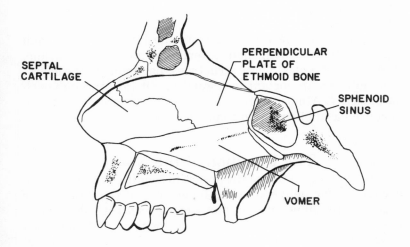

Fig. 2. The nasal septum—a partition composed of bone and cartilage dividing the nose into two cavities of approximately equal size.

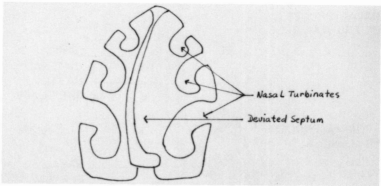

Fig. 3. Deviation of the nasal septum.

The inside of the nose is divided into two approximately equal cavities by a partition called the *nasal septum*. Like the skeleton of the external nose, the lower portion of the septum is formed by cartilage and the upper portion by bone. This skeleton is covered by mucous membrane that lines the entire interior of the nose. Although deviations of the septum (fig. 3) may interfere with nasal breathing, no septum is perfectly straight and thus many septal deviations do not cause symptoms.

Three small bones project from the lateral wall of each nasal cavity and, with their covering of mucous membrane, form the *turbinates*. These structrues, particularly the lowest turbinate, are important in regulating air flow through each nasal cavity. Abnormal function of the turbinates is more apt to cause nasal obstruction than are septal deviations.

The Function of the Nose

The major function of the nose is to condition inhaled air to prepare it for delivery to the lungs so that the delicate air spaces of the lungs are not damaged by contact with atmospheric air. In addition to cleansing, inspired air undergoes warming and humidification from the air stream's contact with the turbinates. The ability of the turbinates to rapidly change their size allows regulation of the amount of heat and moisture provided to inspired air.

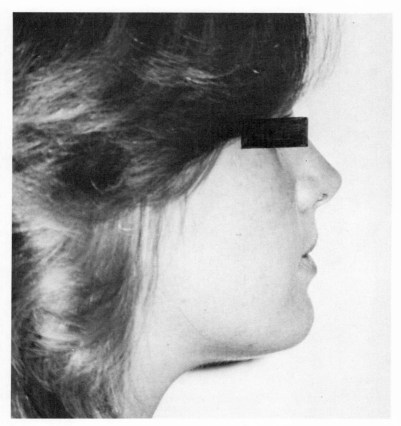

Fig. 4. Convex profile. Note that the tip is located slightly above the plane of the rest of the nose.

Characteristics of the Ideal Nose

Although it is virtually impossible to reshape a nose to exact specifications, the ideal nose has certain characteristics that the surgeon tries to reproduce. The tip is the focal point of the nose. Ideally it should be located slightly above the plane of the remainder of the nose when seen in profile. The shape of the ideal nose in profile is largely a matter of personal preference. Many women prefer a slight slope or convexity while others prefer a straight *dorsum* (fig. 4). Men

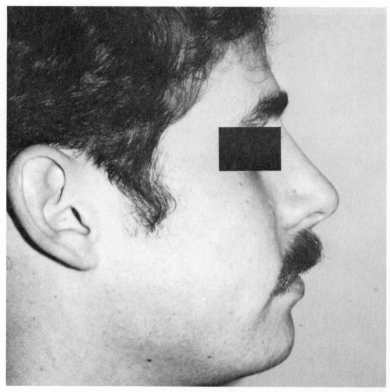

Fig. 5. Straight profile usually preferred by men.

usually prefer a strong, straight profile or a nose with a suggestion of a small hump (fig. 5).

The nasal tip should be relatively thin and delicate and as seen from the base should have the shape of an equilateral triangle. The nostrils should be oval and equal in size.

The angle at which the nose is tilted upward varies with sex and height. The ideal male nose shows an angle of 90–100 degrees between the lip and tip while the female nose has an angle of 100–120 degrees. Taller people require less tilt as shorter people look directly into the nostrils when there is a large angle. Conversely, shorter people can tolerate a greater tilt.

Effects of Aging on the Appearance of the Nose

With increasing age, the tip of the nose gradually falls. This gradual descent actually begins in childhood and continues throughout life. The nose of the infant and child is characteristically "turned up." By adolescence, the angle the tip makes with the upper lip has decreased to 90–100 degrees in the average male and 100–120 degrees in the average female. This position usually lasts into early and mid-adulthood but between forty and fifty gradual descent frequently takes place (fig. 6).

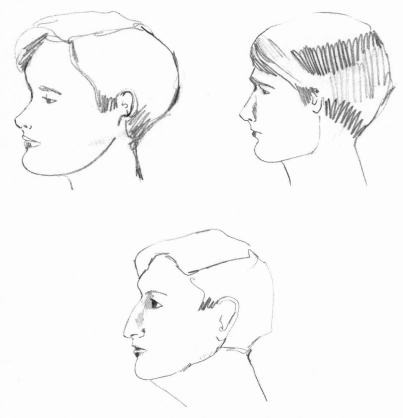

Fig. 6. Changes in the nasal tip that occur with aging.

This drooping of the tip is a consequence of the gradual loosening of the tissue bands that maintain the normal elevated tip against the forces of gravity. Absorption of fat at the base of the nose and the loss of upper teeth and surrounding bone accentuates "tip droop."

As the tip falls, the nose seems longer. The bony skeleton becomes more prominent and frequently a frank hump appears. If a person with such a tip drop elevates the tip with his fingers while looking in a mirror, he will notice that the hump becomes smaller or disappears.

Causes of Nasal Deformities

Nasal deformities fall into two basic categories. Perhaps their most common cause is injury. Such an injury may produce an obvious fracture of the nasal skeleton that heals in an abnormal position and causes a deformity. Some injuries may produce deformities that are not recognizable at the time of injury but develop gradually when scar tissue contracts or new bone proliferates in traumatized areas.

Trauma during childhood may damage growth centers in the nasal skeleton and produce deformities that become apparent only during the long period of growth and maturation of the nose.

The second major group of factors that may cause nasal deformities are congenital problems. This is a broad category that encompasses such possibilities as heredity, toxic or infectious influences during pregnancy, as well as nasal injury during childbirth.

Miscellaneous things such as nasal tumors, disorders of metabolism, or irradiation are sometimes causes of nasal deformities. In the absence of a definite history of nasal injury, hereditary predisposition, or an obvious congenital problem, it may be impossible for the surgeon to determine the actual cause of a nasal deformity.

Nasal deformities, of course, may also be caused by complications after septal surgery or rhinoplasty. Such deformities may be obvious, or so subtle that they are noticeable only to nasal surgeons. The goal of cosmetic nasal surgery is to improve the appearance of the nose while avoiding the telltale "operated-on look."

Selection of Candidates for Rhinoplasty

Candidates for cosmetic nasal surgery are selected by the cosmetic facial surgeon after careful evaluation. Of particular interest is the candidate's description of the exact features of the nose he or she wants corrected. The surgeon will not accept general statements such as "my nose is too big" or "it just doesn't fit my face," but seeks more specific responses, such as dissatisfaction with a hump, a wide tip, or a crooked nose. After all, if a person cannot describe the things about the nose that are most objectionable to him, the surgeon cannot be expected to perform corrective surgery that will satisfy his desires and expectations.

The surgeon next asks whether the candidate has breathing problems or wants surgery for cosmetic reasons only. If nasal obstruction is a problem, he asks further questions to define the nature of this problem. Obstruction that alternates from side to side is suggestive of turbinate abnormalities, while unilateral obstruction is compatible with a septal deviation. Some people are reluctant to request nasal surgery for cosmetic reasons alone and say that they experience breathing difficulty even though they do not. As cosmetic nasal surgery is now widely accepted, this reluctance is unnecessary, it can only cloud the issue, and may even result in unnecessary surgery on the nasal septum. It is important to remember that most septums are not perfectly straight and if the surgeon finds a deviation on the side where the patient complains of an obstruction, he may assume that the deviation is responsible. Some cosmetic surgeons routinely perform septal surgery in conjunction with rhinoplasty on the assumption that asymptomatic deviations may become symptomatic after the shape of the nose is altered. Others, however, do not agree with this.

Questions about nasal disorders such as frequent colds, allergies and nosebleeds are then asked. The general medical condition of the candidate is assessed (see chapter 1).

The emotional makeup of the prospective patient is evaluated. His motives in seeking rhinoplasty are explored (a simple "I want my nose to look better" is often sufficient) and the patient's expectations of surgery are discussed. It is particularly important that these be realistic. The patient must understand that the goal of rhinoplasty is improvement in the appearance of the nose rather than absolute perfection. On occasion, the surgeon may feel uncomfortable with the motivation or general emotional makeup of a patient and may request psychiatric or psychologic evaluation before scheduling surgery. Further details of psychological aspects of cosmetic surgery are discussed in chapter 3.

After this interview, the surgeon examines the nose. The general size and shape of the nose are important in assessing the possible benefits of rhinoplasty, particularly with respect to the wishes and expectations of the patient. Although noses of all configurations may benefit from rhinoplasty, certain types of noses are more amenable to satisfactory surgical results.

Contrary to the popular belief that cosmetic facial surgeons routinely transform unattractive noses into objects of beauty, the surgeon is generally limited by the preoperative structure of the nasal skeleton. This and the thickness and texture of the skin are the most important factors in predicting the postoperative result. This should not be surprising when one considers that in most creative endeavors the result depends to a great extent on the quality of material with which one has to work.

Two other factors interact with this to produce the final nasal appearance. An obvious consideration is the skill of the surgeon. The third factor is the behavior of the nasal tissues during the healing phase that follows the operation.

As a general rule, large noses are more suitable for cosmetic surgery than are small noses. Reduction procedures are technically less difficult than operations designed to increase nasal size as such procedures frequently require the use of fragile bone or cartilage grafts or inert implants. Time frequently alters the size and shape of such grafts and it is not uncommon for implant materials to be rejected by the body.

Noses exhibiting humps in profile are particularly amenable to good results, and patients with such noses are perhaps the most commonly accepted candidates for rhinoplasty.

Noses that look crooked from the front are more difficult to correct, particularly if the deviation is caused by deformity of the cartilaginous part of the nose. Although such deformities may be satisfactorily corrected at end of the operation, postoperative stresses on the cartilage occasionally produce disappointing recurrent deviations despite the best efforts of the surgeon.

Thick-skinned noses may also pose difficult surgical problems as the ability of such skin to contract and adequately drape over the new nasal skeleton is often limited.

Techniques of rhinoplastic surgery have evolved to the point that the competent and experienced nasal surgeon can expect reasonably consistent results in most of the patients he accepts for cosmetic nasal surgery. The prospective patient, however, should be aware that several things that influence the final result are beyond the control of the surgeon. The most important of these are uncertainties in the healing phase and the possibility of minor nasal injury during this period. For these reasons, nasal surgeons generally inform candidates for rhinoplasty that revision procedures are occasionally required to get an optimum result.

The nasal septum and turbinates are then examined to see if there are structural abnormalities that may produce breathing difficulties preoperatively or after rhinoplasty.

As the goal of rhinoplasty is to produce a nose that is in harmony with the rest of the face, this operation is frequently performed in conjunction with procedures designed to modify other aspects of the face. The most common such procedure is augmentation of the chin, accomplished by insertion of an inert implant beneath the skin overlying the prominence of the chin (see chapter 15). The surgeon will analyze the facial profile to determine whether such a correction would be beneficial.

Occasionally the chin weakness of a patient may be great enough to warrant a procedure involving advancement of part of the lower jaw for correction of the deformity. Patients with deficient facial profiles caused by dental abnormalities may also benefit from such procedures, as may people with excessively prominent chins.

Getting Ready for Rhinoplasty

The prospective patient is carefully counselled about the operation and the postoperative period. Possible complications are carefully explained.

Photographs are taken and discussed with the patient. The areas to be corrected are identified and associated defects and asymmetries the patient may not be aware of that will not be affected by rhinoplasty are pointed out.

The goals and limitations of rhinoplasty are reviewed. Possible complications of the operation are discussed and an informed consent agreement is signed.

Fees for rhinoplasty are usually paid in advance, and a member of the surgeon's office staff generally discusses them with the patient before scheduling the surgery (see chapter 1).

The patient is told not to use aspirin for at least one week before surgery as it may interfere with blood clotting and result in increased operative or postoperative bleeding. Instructions are also given regarding the use of other medications that he may be taking.

Final Preparations for Rhinoplasty

Rhinoplasty may be performed either in a hospital operating room or an outpatient surgical facility (see chapter 5). If it is scheduled in a hospital, the patient is usually admitted on the evening before for preoperative examinations and laboratory tests. Patients undergoing surgery in outpatient facilities arrive at least one hour before surgery. They are usually instructed to avoid food for six to eight hours before surgery to minimize the chance of vomiting.

Preoperative Medication

Sedatives may be given by mouth several hours before surgery and reinforced with injections one hour before.

Anesthesia for Rhinoplasty

Although some surgeons perform rhinoplasty under general anesthesia, most such operations are performed under local anesthesia, obtained by injection of anesthetic solution into the nasal tissues.

If surgery is to be performed under general anesthesia, an anesthetist will administer the appropriate anesthetic.

The Operation

Most rhinoplasty procedures are performed through incisions placed on the inside of the nose so that there are no external scars. In some cases, small external incisions are used, usually to reduce the size and flare of the nostrils. After maturation, these scars are usually inconspicuous. Some surgeons prefer to use other external incisions when performing rhinoplasty on a very deformed nose, but such incisions are placed where they will be relatively unnoticed after healing. If there are symptomatic deviations of the nasal septum, they are usually corrected before reshaping the outside of the nose.

The skin is elevated from the underlying bone and cartilage, and, using specially designed instruments, the surgeon modifies the nasal skeleton. Reshaping the bone requires making controlled fractures that produce postoperative swelling and discoloration of the nose and eyes. After the procedure is completed, the skin redrapes over the new nasal skeleton (fig. 7). Light gauze packing is put inside the nose to prevent bleeding, and an external tape dressing is applied. A small plaster splint is fashioned to fit the nose (fig. 8).

The Postoperative Period

After completion of the operation, cold compresses are applied to the nose and eyes for twenty-four hours to minimize swelling and discoloration. The patient is told to remain in bed with his head elevated to further minimize swelling. The degree of swelling and discoloration varies, depending to a large extent on the thickness of the patient's bone and nasal skin as well as to his normal reaction to injury.

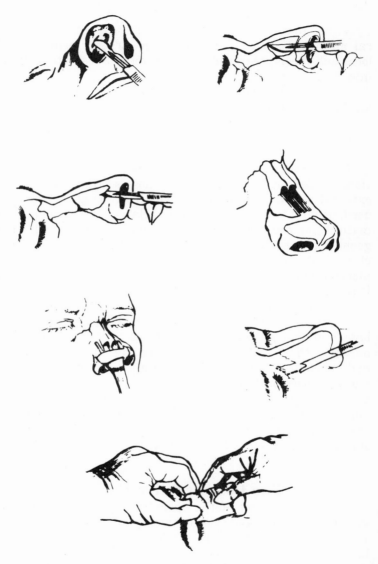

*Fig. 7. Steps in performing rhinoplasty: Intranasal incision,
elevation of skin from the cartilage bone, removal of the
cartilaginous portion of the hump, removal of the boney hump using
a chisel, fracture of the nasal bones using a chisel (ostotome).*

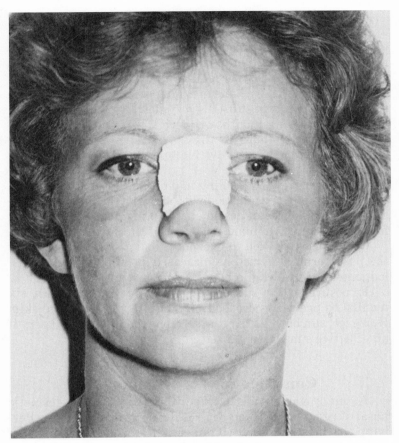

Fig. 8. Plaster cast in place after rhinoplasty.

If the operation was performed in a hospital, the patient is usually discharged the morning after surgery. The gauze packing is usually removed at this time. Some surgeons, however, prefer to leave this packing in longer if extensive septal surgery was necessary.

The patient is told to continue applying cold compresses until twenty-four hours after the operation and to sleep with the head of his bed elevated for several weeks to encourage resolution of swelling. Pain is not usually severe after rhinoplasty, and it is readily controlled with mild analgesics.

Five to seven days after surgery the cast and tape dressing are removed. This unveiling, often characterized dramatically by Hollywood, is frequently a moment of relative disappointment for the patient as he sees a nose that is somewhat swollen. Although 90 percent of this swelling has usually resolved by the end of the second postoperative week, the remaining 10 percent subsides very slowly and complete resolution may take six months or more. The patient should also be aware that changes in the appearance of the nose may occur during the ensuing twelve to eighteen months as scar tissue maturates.

After resolution of swelling and discoloration, the surgeon may recommend consultation with a cosmetologist for instruction in the use of cosmetics and hairstyling to minimize minor facial defects and to make the most of the surgery.

Care must be taken to prevent minor nasal injury during the postoperative period as increased swelling and even dislodgement of the fragile bones can occur.

Exposure to the sun should be avoided for at least six months to prevent increased pigmentation of the nasal skin. However, sun bathing is permitted one month after surgery if an effective sunscreen is used.

Complications of Rhinoplasty

As many variables can affect the final result of cosmetic nasal surgery, unsatisfactory results occasionally occur. Perhaps the most common complication is the development of fullness in the area just above the nasal tip. This fullness is frequently related to accumulation of scar tissue there and is called a "polly beak" or "parrot's beak" because of the appearance of the nasal profile. This problem is more common after rhinoplasty performed on large noses and on noses with thick skin. In some cases, this deformity is accentuated by a gradual drop or settling of the tip toward the face. If detected early, many polly beaks can be eliminated by a series of injections of cortisonelike material into the area. This substance is very effective in reducing scar tissue. Polly beaks that do not respond to this treatment, or those due to other things besides excessive accumulation of scar tissue are treated by revision surgery that is usually delayed until at least one year after the primary procedure.

Excessive removal of nasal bone may produce a "ski jump" profile, and excessive shortening of the nose can result in a "pig snout" deformity. Excessive removal of the cartilages of the nasal tip may produce irregularities or pinching of the tip. These problems, however, do not usually occur after rhinoplasty performed by an experienced surgeon.

On occasion, a small residual nasal hump may appear after swelling is resolved. This is more common after removal of a large hump, or in a nose with thick skin. If this hump is objectionable, it can be easily removed by a revision operation.

Surgery of a crooked nose presents a particular challenge to the cosmetic facial surgeon. Even with the most experienced surgeons, residual deviation can occur postoperatively, particularly if the preoperative deviation was secondary to abnormalities of the cartilaginous part of the nose. The person with a crooked nose is carefully warned about this preoperatively. Revision operations can be performed in an attempt to correct such deviations, but complete resolution is sometimes not obtained.

Bleeding may occur in the early postoperative period and is usually easily controlled by pinching the tip with the fingers for ten minutes. If bleeding is persistent, however, nasal packing may have to be reinserted.

Nasal obstruction sometimes occurs after cosmetic nasal surgery. Breathing difficulty during the early postoperative period may be secondary to swelling or may be the result of a concurrent upper respiratory infection or allergy. Persistent nasal obstruction may be a consequence of a septal deviation or abnormality of the turbinates that may require further treatment. As noted, some surgeons routinely remove septal deviations during rhinoplasty on the assumption that these areas may become symptomatic after the size of the nose is reduced.

Infection is a rare complication of rhinoplasty but it can be devastating if it occurs. It is more common if the surgery is performed while the patient has a cold or an exacerbation of an allergy. It is also more likely to occur if the operation is

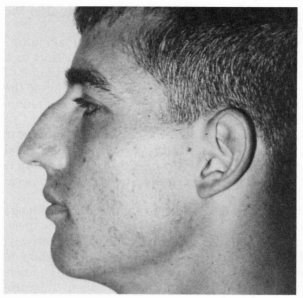

Fig. 9.
Preoperative
photo of male
patient.

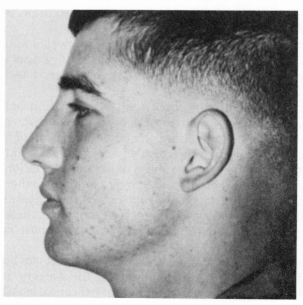

Fig. 10.
Postoperative
photo of same
patient.

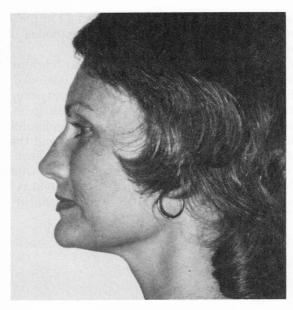

*Fig. 11.
Preoperative
photo of female
patient.*

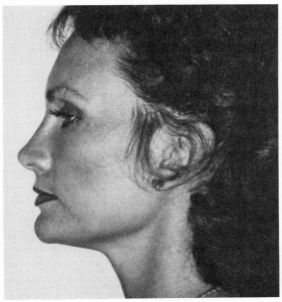

*Fig. 12.
Postoperative
photo of same
patient.*

performed when there is superficial skin infection ("pimple") on or near the nose. For this reason, surgery is postponed if any of these conditions are present.

This impressive list of possible complications may frighten the candidate for cosmetic nasal surgery. It should be stressed, however, that the most serious of these are unlikely to occur when the operation is performed by an experienced surgeon. Such surgeons have a thorough knowledge of the mechanics and dynamics of this complex operation and understand the basic factors that tend to produce undesirable results. Techniques of rhinoplastic surgery have evolved to the point that the experienced surgeon can expect reasonably consistent results in most of the patients he *accepts* for cosmetic nasal surgery (figs. 12, 13, 14, 15).

15

Correcting the Chin

The position of the chin is of prime importance to the facial profile. It functions in concert with the forehead and nose in determining facial balance and harmony. Analysis of profiles has shown that in the ideal face, the chin is tangential to a line connecting the root of the nose and a point just behind the anterior border of the upper lip (fig. 1). The ideal chin position can also be estimated by a line dropped perpendicular to the border of the lower lip. The ideal chin is at a tangent to this line.

Chin abnormalities are of two basic types. Perhaps the most common is underdevelopment or "weakness" of the chin (*microgenia*). Such weakness is usually slight but occurs in various degrees (fig. 2).

Overdevelopment of the chin is called *macrogenia* and also occurs in various degrees (fig. 3).

Abnormalities of the chin are often accompanied by abnormalities of the jaws and teeth resulting in *malocclusion* (see chapter 16) that may impair the chewing mechanism. Chin weakness associated with underdevelopment of the lower jaw is called *retrognathia*, while prominence associated with overdevelopment of the jaw is called *prognathism*.

Recession or protrusion of the chin is also frequently asso-

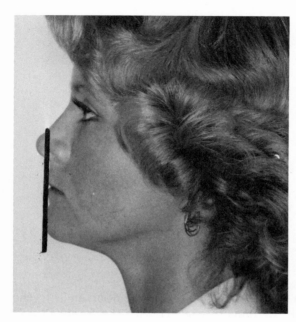

Fig. 1. The "ideal" chin lies on a tangent to the line described in the text.

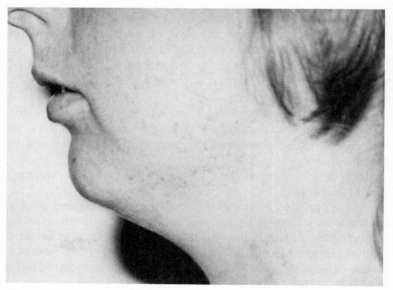

Fig. 2. "Weakness" of the chin.

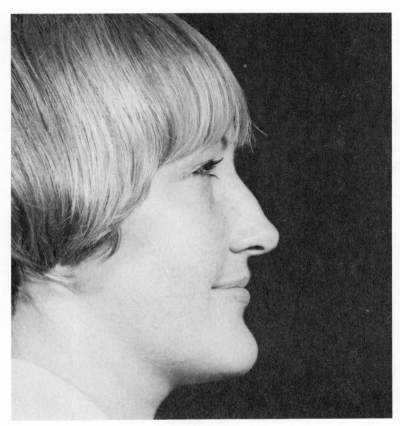

Fig. 3. Prominence of the chin.

ciated with abnormalities in the position of the lips. People
with weak chins are often unable to keep their lips completely
closed without strain. People with protruding chins frequently
have a lower lip that overlaps the upper lip and produces a
"bulldog" appearance.

Stereotyped personality characteristics have been popu-
larly associated with chin abnormalities. People with protruding chins are often thought of as stubborn and belligerent,
while those with receding chins are considered weak or cow-
ardly. There is, of course, no evidence to suggest that these
stereotypes have any significance whatsoever.

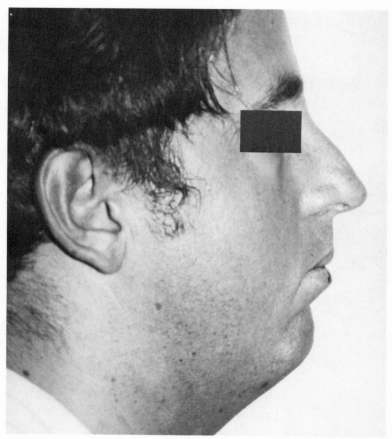

Fig. 4. Chin "weakness" associated with a forehead that slopes back and a prominent nose. Note the double chin.

The position of the chin often enhances or exaggerates other abnormalities of the facial profile. The combination of a forehead that slopes backwards and a receding chin, for example, produces a "birdlike" appearance (fig. 4). A small chin makes a large nose appear more prominent, while a protruding chin creates the illusion of a smaller nose. For this reason, correction of the chin is often done in conjunction with cosmetic nasal surgery (fig. 5).

As chin recession also affects the chin-neck angle (see

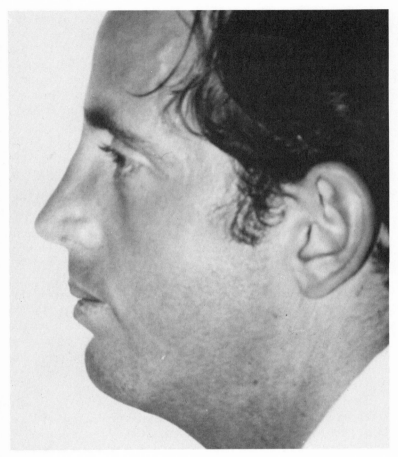

Fig. 5. Improvement following rhinoplasty and chin augmentation.

chapter 15) and so may accentuate sagging skin and fat accumulation (double chin) in this region, correction is often recommended as an adjunct to face-lift surgery.

Diagnosis and Evaluation of Chin Abnormalities

While the presence of an abnormal chin is usually obvious, many people are unaware of small abnormalities, especially mild degrees of recession. When evaluating a patient for cosmetic facial surgery, the surgeon scrutinizes the entire facial profile. In some cases he finds a chin abnormality that significantly affects facial harmony and balance. As correction of this abnormality in conjunction with other cosmetic procedures may substantially improve the patient's final appearance, the cosmetic surgeon is justified in pointing it out to him—even if he had not previously been aware of it.

Most cosmetic surgeons find that as many as 15 to 25 percent of candidates for cosmetic nasal surgery would benefit from chin augmentation. This figure is somewhat lower for candidates for the face-lift operation.

The surgeon's findings on examining the facial profile are confirmed by studying photographs of the candidate. The degree of chin recession or protrusion can be analyzed, and the benefits expected of correction demonstrated to the prospective patient.

As abnormalities of chin position are often accompanied by *dental malocclusion*, the cosmetic surgeon searches for this before recommending surgery. If significant dental malformation is present, orthodontic or surgical correction of the dental abnormality (see chapter 16—*Orthognathic Surgery*) may be advised. If, on the other hand, significant malocclusion is not present, attention can be focused entirely on the cosmetic abnormality produced by the chin recession or protrusion.

If dental problems are noted, the patient is frequently referred to an oral surgeon or orthodontist for further evaluation. These specialists examine the teeth and jaws and analyze dental and facial relationships by studying special X rays called *cephalometric radiographs*. Plaster models of the teeth and jaws may also help to plan appropriate treatment (see chapter 16).

Methods of Correcting
Chin Abnormalities—Receding Chin

Mild to moderate degrees of chin recession can be corrected by placing a graft or implant beneath the skin over the chin prominence. In the past, grafts of living bone or cartilage were recommended, but since the development of artificial

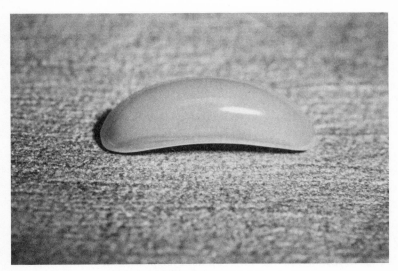

Fig. 6. Silicone rubber chin implant.

implants of medical grade silicone, this material is used by most surgeons because of its convenience and reliability. These silicone implants may be preformed or may be carved to the desired size by the surgeon during the operation. Bone and cartilage grafts frequently decrease in size over the years because they are gradually absorbed.

Chin implants (fig. 6) can be placed through incisions in the skin just beneath the chin or an incision inside the lower lip (fig. 7). An advantage of the lip incision is that it leaves no external scars. Some surgeons, however, feel that the rate of infections around implants is higher with this approach (others disagree) and prefer to use the skin incision. The resulting scar is usually relatively inconspicuous.

Moderate degrees of recession can also be treated by an operation in which the bone forming the chin is cut below the roots of the teeth and moved forward to increase its prominence (fig. 8). The bone is held in this position with wires during the healing period. Severe degrees of chin recession are frequently corrected in this manner because large implants are associated with more postoperative complications than smaller ones.

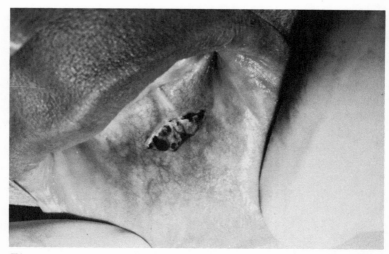

Fig. 7. Incision inside lower lip used for placement of chin implant.

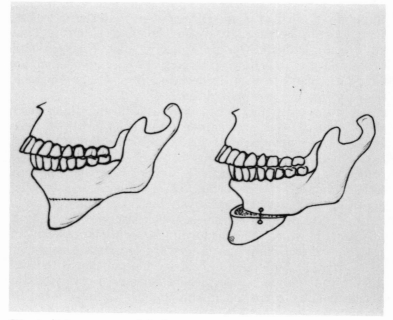

Fig. 8. Advancement of the lower portion of the mandible.

If significant malocclusion of the teeth is associated with chin recession, the entire front segment of the lower jaw may be advanced to correct both dental and cosmetic problems. This procedure is discussed in more detail in chapter 16.

Correcting Excessive Chin Prominence

Correction of chin prominence requires more extensive surgery than does chin augmentation. Several operations are available.

If dental occlusion is normal, the chin can be reduced in size by removing the prominent portion. Some surgeons prefer to excise a segment of bone from this area and slide the chin back, again using wires to maintain position during healing (figs. 9 and 10). These procedures can be done through

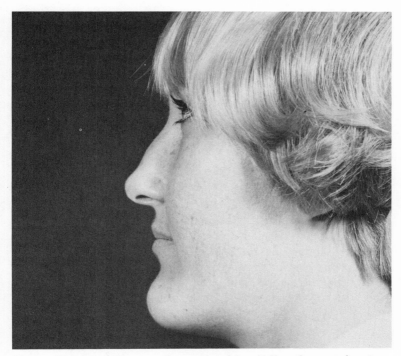

Fig. 9. Chin prominence to be corrected by sliding the prominent portion of the mandible backwards.

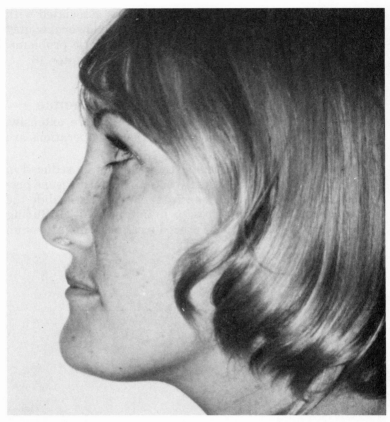

Fig. 10. Results of the operation.

incisions placed in the skin beneath the chin or in the mouth.

If chin prominence is associated with dental malocclusion, the entire lower jaw may be placed in a more posterior position. Operations for such a correction are described in chapter 16. Orthodontic treatment may be recommended in conjunction with any of these surgical procedures.

Preparation for Surgery

As these procedures are frequently performed in conjunction with other cosmetic operations, preparation is similar to that described for those procedures. Proper dental hygiene is important before surgery on the jaws. If incisions are to be placed in the mouth, the patient may be instructed to brush the teeth with an antiseptic soap on the day before surgery.

If external incisions are to be used, the location and extent of the scars that will result is discussed, and the process of wound healing and scar maturation is reviewed with the patient.

Possible complications of the operation are discussed and an informed consent agreement giving the surgeon permission to perform the surgery is signed.

Complications of Chin Correction

Complications of chin augmentation or reduction vary with procedure employed. If artificial chin implants are used, the possibility of infection requiring removal of the implant must be considered. After this foreign material is removed, such an infection can be readily controlled with antibiotics, and, if the patient wants the implant replaced, it can be at a later date. Frequently, however, a satisfactory amount of augmentation is obtained by the formation of scar tissue beneath the skin.

In some cases, artificial implants have gradually eroded the bone of the chin, making recession recur. This is less apt to happen if the implant is placed on top of the membrane that nourishes the bone (*periosteum*) rather than below this membrane.

On occasion, a chin implant becomes slightly displaced during healing and, as a result, feels somewhat crooked beneath the skin. Although this may initially worry the patient, in most instances the appearance of the chin is not altered. Unless the chin actually looks unnatural, there is little to be gained by attempting to reposition the implant. Patients are instructed to avoid manipulating this area.

Operations for realigning bone or teeth may also be complicated by infection. If such infection cannot be readily controlled with antibiotics, early removal of wires may be required. This may result in incomplete healing of the bone, causing abnormal mobility, and necessitate an additional operation to achieve complete bony union.

In some cases, the chin correction wanted may fall short of expectation when major shifts of the jaw are involved. But, because of its profound effect on facial balance and harmony, surgical correction of the chin is one of the most satisfying and rewarding cosmetic facial operations.

16

Orthognathic Surgery

The lower third of the face plays an important role in total facial balance and harmony. The skeleton of this portion of the face consists of the upper and lower jaws (*maxilla* and *mandible*) and, as in other areas, this skeleton is important in determining surface configuration. Surgical correction of deformities of the jaws and associated teeth is called *orthognathic* surgery (*ortho*—straight or normal; *gnathos*—jaw). It has developed into an important part of cosmetic facial surgery.

Orthognathic surgery, however, is rarely performed solely for cosmetic reasons. Deformities of the jaws are usually accompanied by abnormalities in their function and so the goals of orthognathic surgery are improvement of both function and appearance. Interestingly, surveys of patients who have undergone orthognathic surgery show that they tend to be more pleased by improvements in their appearance and self-image than by their bite.

Types of Deformities That Can Be Corrected by Orthognathic Surgery

Many abnormalities of jaw appearance and function are treatable by orthognathic surgery. One of the most common conditions amenable to surgical correction is prognathism of the mandible, which makes the lower jaw abnormally prominent (fig. 1). Excessive protrusion of the maxilla (*maxillary prognathism*) is less common (fig. 2). In some cases, both the maxilla and mandible are protuberant—a condition called *bimaxillary prognathism* (fig. 3).

Abnormal recession of the mandible, called *mandibular retrognathia* (fig. 4) and underdevelopment of the maxilla (*maxillary retrognathia*) are other conditions that orthognathic surgery may be used to correct.

Occasionally a patient has no actual recession of either jaw, but develops an abnormal tilt of one or both jaws resulting in an inability to close the front teeth—a condition called open bite or *apertognathia*.

It must be stressed that satisfactory correction of these deformities is rarely possible by orthognathic surgery alone. The surgeon must work closely with the orthodontist to properly diagnose and plan treatment. Orthodontic treatment is usually necessary to properly align abnormal teeth before surgery and is sometimes necessary to maintain correction after surgery. In no way should orthognathic surgery be thought of as a substitute for orthodontics.

Some jaw deformities, however, such as *macrogenia* and *microgenia*, are not associated with abnormalities of the teeth and they can be corrected without altering the teeth. In macrogenia, only the portion of the mandible that forms the chin is enlarged, causing excessive chin prominence. Underdevelopment of the chin without the characteristic dental abnormalities of retrognathia is called microgenia.

Cosmetic Defects Associated with Jaw Deformities

The consequences of enlargement or underdevelopment of the upper and lower jaws are obvious. Enlargement of the mandible (prognathism or microgenia) produces excessive protrusion of the chin and often results in a belligerent or "bulldog" appearance. Underdevelopment of the mandible (retrognathia or microgenia) produces the "weak chin" or "Andy Gump" profile.

Overdevelopment of the maxilla may also give the illusion

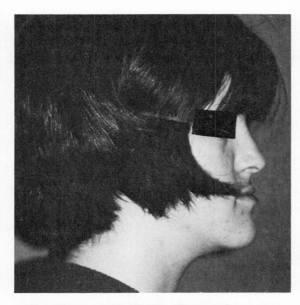

Fig. 1.
Prominence of
the mandible
(prognathism).

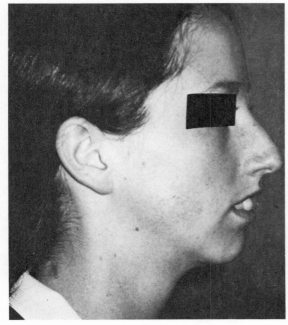

Fig. 2.
Excessive
protrusion of the
upper jaw
(maxilla)
associated with
recession of the
mandible
(mandibular
retrognathia).

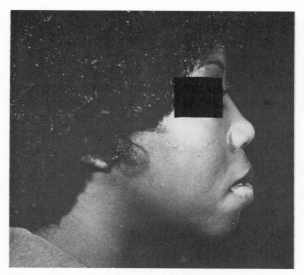

Fig. 3. Excessive protrusion of both maxilla and mandible (bimaxillary protrusion).

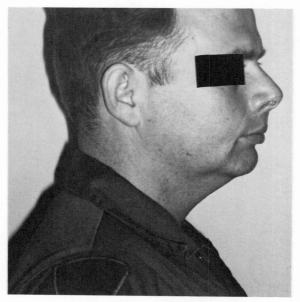

Fig. 4. Recession of the mandible (mandibular retrognathia).

of chin weakness but it produces "buck teeth" too. Under-development of the maxilla may produce an illusion of chin prominence associated with a "dish face" appearance.

These skeletal deformities are also responsible for an ab-normal appearance of the lips. In mandibular prognathism the lower lip is protruding and assumes a pouting position. The lower lip is displaced backwards in mandibular retro-gnathia and it is often difficult to keep the lips closed without strain. The chin often appears flat instead of rounded. Be-cause the upper limb of the chin–neck angle (see chapter 15) is shortened, this angle may appear less acute, producing a "double chin."

People with maxillary prognathism often have "short" up-per lips and show an excessive amount of upper gum when they smile.

Dental Abnormalities and Jaw Deformities

Some abnormalities of the teeth associated with jaw de-formities are obvious, such as the "buck teeth" from over-development of the maxilla. Other abnormalities of the teeth are not readily noticeable, but cause problems for those people affected. For example, some people with large degrees of mandibular or maxillary overdevelopment complain that they cannot bite into sandwiches because their front teeth do not come together.

Many dental complications of jaw deformities are dor-mant until later. Persistent abnormal occlusion of the teeth often produces malfunction of the jaw joint and the muscles responsible for chewing. This often causes discomfort in the region of the ear appearing as early as adolescence. Diseases of the gums are more common in patients with deformities of the jaw, as is premature loss of teeth. Jaw deformities often make it difficult to fit dentures.

Causes of Jaw Deformities

Most jaw deformities are the consequence of heredity or of the interaction of genetic predisposition with environmental factors during growth and development. Many of these environmental factors are obscure. Controversy surrounds the role of such things as thumbsucking, abnormal swallowing patterns ("tongue thrusting"), and chronic mouth breathing in contributing to these abnormalities. Direct injury to the jaws during development is an obvious cause of deformities.

History of Orthognathic Surgery

As did many other forms of cosmetic surgery, orthognathic surgery originated in the mid-nineteenth century. In 1846 an American dental surgeon described an operation for correction of mandibular prognathism. Although this procedure received some attention and stimulated other surgeons to devise improved methods for correction of this abnormality, little effort was made to correct other jaw deformities until the early twentieth century. At that time a series of operations to correct all types of deformities was devised by European surgeons.

It was not until after World War II that American surgeons again showed interest in these operations. Thanks to the efforts of oral surgeons, there has been a surge of interest in these procedures since that time.

Contemporary surgeons use sophisticated methods to diagnose jaw deformities and have at their disposal several alternate procedures for correcting each deformity. Advances in anesthesia, pre- and postoperative care, antibiotics for control of infections, and the availability of expert orthodontic management have facilitated the enormous growth of orthognathic surgery.

Diagnosis of Jaw Deformities

While the presence of a jaw deformity is usually suggested by the appearance of the lower third of the face, an exact diagnosis of the nature of the deformity requires further study.

Careful examination of the jaws, teeth, and lips, supplemented by study of medical photographs of the full face and facial profile, generally provides a basic idea of the deformity.

Exact diagnosis, however, depends on evaluation of special X rays and plaster models of the teeth. The patient in figure 4, for example, shows an obvious weakness of the chin. The first impression of a casual observer might be that this weakness is a result of underdevelopment of the mandible (mandibular retrognathia). This deformity, however, could also be a consequence of an overdeveloped maxilla (maxillary prognathism) or underdeveloped chin (microgenia) without the associated dental abnormalities of retrognathia. Similarly, prominence of the chin, although usually secondary to mandibular prognathism, may be a consequence of maxillary retrognathia or macrogenia.

Special X ray examination of the skull with a technique called *cephalometrics* is of value in resolving diagnostic questions that arise after examining a patient and studying his photographs. An X ray of the skull in profile forms the basis for cephalometric analysis. This X ray differs from a routine skull X ray in that the head is placed in a standard position so that measurement and comparison with other cephalometrograms can be made. The X ray not only shows bony detail of the jaws and teeth, it shows the soft tissue profile of the chin and lips.

A series of lines are drawn between fixed points on the X ray, and various angles are formed at their intersections (fig. 5). By comparing these angles with standard values derived from studying the normal population, the surgeon can determine whether the cause of the deformity lies in the mandible or maxilla (or both).

The next diagnostic step is to study plaster models of the patient's dental arches and teeth (fig. 6). These casts are made from molds that form exact impressions of the teeth. The abnormal relationships of the maxillary and mandibular teeth must be determined to plan treatment, and this step is also helpful in determining the extent or limits of possible correction.

Orthodontic consultation is helpful in further defining abnormal relationships of the teeth and jaws. It is often recommended that teeth be properly aligned before surgery so that the patient can obtain maximum benefit from the operation. In some cases, orthodontic treatment is deferred until after

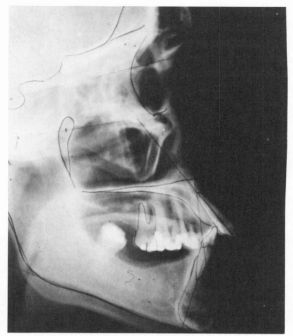

Fig. 5. Cephalometric X ray.

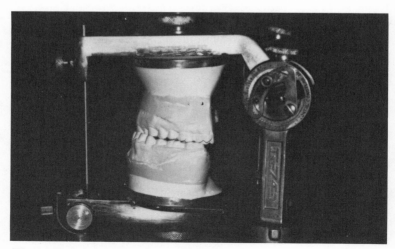

Fig. 6. Dental models.

surgery, and, in others, treatment may be necessary both before and after the operation.

Selection of Candidates for Surgery

Assuming that a candidate for orthognatic surgery has a correctable deformity (as determined by the methods of evaluation described) perhaps the most important considerations in the surgeon's decision to accept the patient are the patient's motives and expectations. Orthognathic surgery is undoubtedly the most rigorous form of cosmetic facial surgery. The pre- and postoperative courses may be prolonged, somewhat uncomfortable, and may entail personal sacrifice. The patient's motivation must be firm, and his personality must be strong enough to withstand sacrifices. It is especially important that expectations, particularly regarding the limitations of the operation, be realistic. When the surgeon is unsure of the patient's personality makeup, psychiatric evaluation may be suggested before accepting the patient (see chapter 3).

Significantly, surveys of patients who have undergone orthognathic surgery show that most are pleased with the results and would undergo these operations again to obtain the desired correction.

Motivation and expectation in relation to cosmetic surgery are discussed in chapter 3. As in all elective surgery, the surgeon will determine that all serious medical problems are under control. He will also determine that the facial skeleton has stopped growing. If orthognathic surgery is performed before this, the deformity is likely to recur as growth continues.

Preparation for Orthognathic Surgery

After accepting a patient for orthognathic surgery, the details of the surgical procedure and postoperative period—including what is expected of the patient—are carefully discussed. If an external incision is planned, the location of the incision and the process of wound healing and scar maturation is discussed (see chapter 7) with the patient. The patient is given a chance to ask questions. Because of the magnitude of orthognathic surgery, the person who is to undergo it should be sure that he thoroughly understands the procedure. Poor preoperative preparation can lead to misunderstanding and disappointment during the postoperative period.

After discussing the procedure, the possible complications and alternative methods of treatment, an informed consent agreement is signed giving the surgeon permission to perform the operation.

Before scheduling the operation, the surgeon will treat any dental infections or other conditions of the mouth or gums that could compromise the surgical result. In some cases, this will entail filling cavities or even pulling teeth. Instructions for dental hygiene will be provided.

If the patient is taking medication, instruction will be provided regarding doses before surgery. Aspirin should be avoided for at least one week as it may cause bleeding during the operation and postoperative period.

Before performing the operation, the surgeon generally plans the surgical correction on the dental casts he has studied, determining that the proposed operation will produce the desired results. The patient usually enters the hospital on the day before surgery to undergo preoperative examinations and laboratory tests.

Anesthesia for Orthognathic Surgery

Most orthognathic surgery is performed under general anesthesia (see chapter 4). Hospitalization is usually required.

The Operative Procedure

The goal of orthognathic surgery is improvement of the appearance of the lower third of the face by advancement or posterior displacement of an abnormal upper or lower jaw, at the same time maintaining or establishing the normal relationship between the upper and lower teeth. Several surgical procedures are available to correct each deformity, but only the most commonly used operations will be discussed.

MANDIBULAR PROGNATHISM

Posterior displacement of the mandible can be accomplished by cutting the toothless portion of the mandible (*ramus*) in a vertical direction and sliding the tooth-bearing portion backward (fig. 7). The fracture line is then approximated with wires and further stabilized by wiring the upper and lower teeth together with appliances (arch bars) that are connected to the teeth (fig. 8). This process is called *inter-*

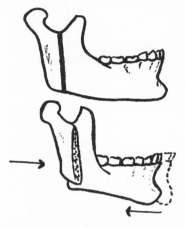

Fig. 7. Vertical ramus osteotomy for correction of mandibular prognathism.

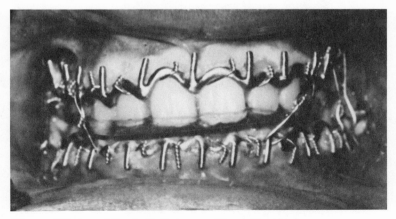

Fig. 8. Wiring of the teeth (intermaxillary fixation).

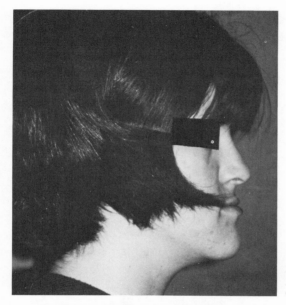

*Fig. 9.
Correction of
mandibular
prognathism,
preoperative
appearance.*

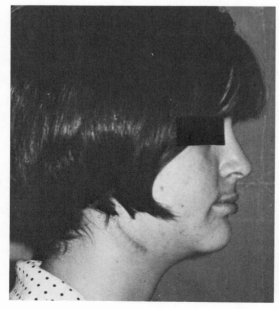

*Fig. 10.
Appearance
several weeks
after surgery.
Note healing scar.*

maxillary fixation (IMF). Although an approach using an incision inside the mouth has been described, the mandible is usually approached through a small skin incision made just below the prominence of the jaw (figs. 9 and 10).

The mandible can also be displaced posteriorly by removing a section of bone from its tooth-bearing portion. As extraction of a tooth is necessary and potential complications are greater, the ramus procedure is preferred by most surgeons. Pre- and postoperative results of an operation to correct mandibular prognathism are shown in figures 9 and 10.

MANDIBULAR RETROGNATHIA

Advancement of the mandible, required for correction of this condition, can be accomplished by surgery of the ramus. A common operation is the C-osteotomy in which a C-shaped cut is made in the ramus and the anterior segment advanced. It is maintained in this position by wiring of the fragments (fig. 11). Additional stabilization is provided by intermaxillary fixation. This procedure is performed through a skin incision like the one used in surgery for prognathism.

Another operation advocated for correction of this deformity is the *sagittal split.* The ramus is approached through an incision in the mouth. The inner surface is separated from the outer surface, enabling the tooth-bearing segment to be advanced anteriorly (fig. 12).

Correction of mandibular retrognathism is illustrated in figures 13 and 14.

MAXILLARY PROTRUSION

This deformity is corrected by removing a segment of bone from the maxilla and sliding the protruberant portion back (fig. 15). Stabilization is also maintained by wiring and intermaxillary fixation. The operation is performed through an incision made in the mouth. Correction of maxillary protrusion is shown in figure 10.

MAXILLARY RETROGNATHIA

In order to correct this deformity, the entire maxilla is separated from its superior attachments and advanced an-

Fig. 11. C-*osteotomy of the mandible.*

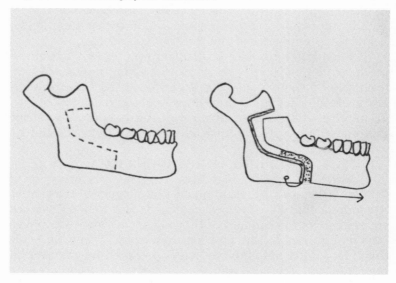

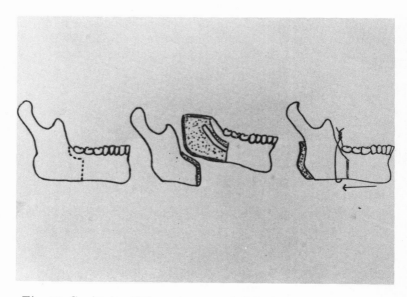

Fig. 12. Sagittal splitting osteotomy of the mandible.

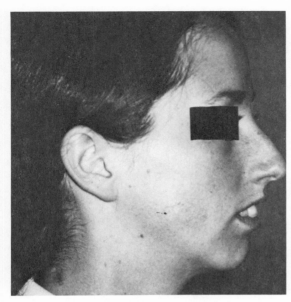

Fig. 13.
Correction of
mandibular
retrognathia
with
simultaneous
correction of
slight maxillary
protrusion
(preoperative
view).

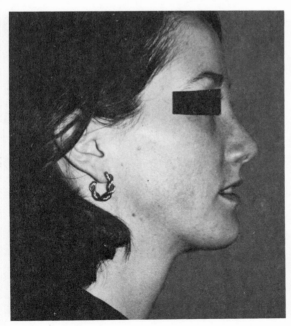

Fig. 14.
Postoperative
result. Patient
also underwent
cosmetic nasal
surgery.

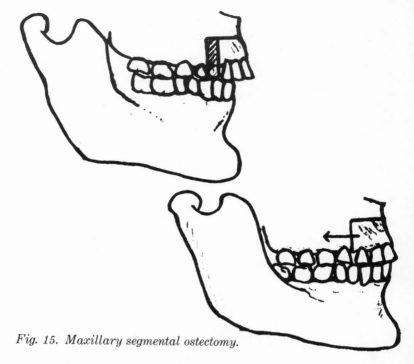

Fig. 15. Maxillary segmental ostectomy.

teriorly, a procedure called a *LeFort I osteotomy* (fig. 16). Again, stabilization is achieved by direct wiring and IMF.

Surgical Correction of the Chin

Mild to moderate deficiencies of the chin without associated abnormalities of the teeth are often corrected by placing silicone rubber implants beneath the skin (see chapter 15). The correction may also be made by separating the bone responsible for the chin prominence and advancing it anteriorly (fig. 17). The bone is maintained in this position by direct wiring. This operation (*horizontal sliding osteotomy*) is usually performed through an incision in the mouth. As this procedure is more involved than chin augmentation with an implant, most patients who want a small correction prefer an implant. The mandibular operation, however, may be more satisfactory for people with greater chin weakness.

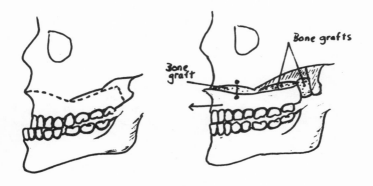

Fig. 16. LeFort I osteotomy.

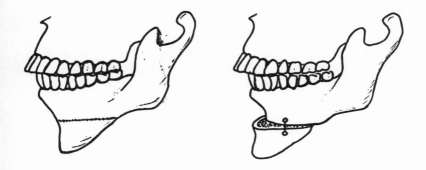

Fig. 17. Horizontal sliding osteotomy for correction of microgenia.

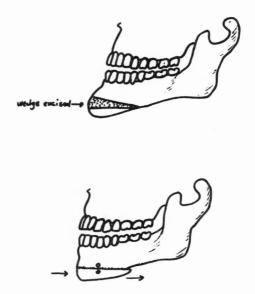

Fig. 18. Horizontal ostectomy for correction of macrogenia.

Excessive chin prominence not accompanied by dental abnormalities may be corrected in two ways. The most direct method consists of simply excising the prominent bone and sculpting a new chin with special bone-cutting instruments (*reduction genioplasty*). The second method involves separating the bone forming the chin prominence from the tooth-bearing portion of the mandible, removing a portion of this bone, and replacing the remaining bone in a more backward position with direct wiring (fig. 18). An advantage of this procedure is that a chin prominence does not have to be sculpted.

In contrast to other forms of orthognathic surgery, the procedures for reducing chin size have a significant rate of failure, as the soft tissue overlying the chin is often not displaced as far back as the bone. Thus prominence may recur due to accumulation of scar tissue. The result of reduction of genioplasty is shown in figure 10, chapter 15.

The Postoperative Period

After the operation, the patient is transferred to a recovery area where his pulse, blood pressure, and breathing are carefully monitored until he is alert. He is then returned to his hospital room where he remains until discharge—usually on the second or third postoperative day. The head of his bed is elevated and cold compresses may also be applied to minimize swelling. Some surgeons prescribe cortisone-like medication to retard further swelling.

Postoperative pain is usually not severe, and medicine is given to ease it. As the teeth are held together by elastic bands or wires, the patient's speech is somewhat muffled. As he adjusts, his speech improves and becomes easy to understand.

Vomiting is an important danger in the early postoperative period. As the patient's teeth are wired, vomiting could result in entry of this material into the lungs, causing pneumonia. Medicine is administered at the first sign of nausea, and, as an additional safeguard, scissors and wirecutters are placed at the bedside so that the elastic bands or wires holding the teeth together can immediately be cut if vomiting occurs. Fortunately, this is unusual.

Dental wiring also makes it difficult to provide adequate nutrition. During the first twenty-four postoperative hours, an intravenous line is in place. After its removal the patient is taught to take liquids without opening his mouth. He takes commercial high caloric liquids, and liquids prepared from solid food with a blender, during the six to eight weeks of intermaxillary fixation that follow most orthognathic surgery. In spite of this, the average patient loses ten to twenty pounds.

Cleaning the teeth and gums is an important task during intermaxillary fixation. Before discharge from the hospital, the patient is taught to use mouth cleansers frequently and is instructed in proper methods of cleaning the teeth and gums.

If small rubber drains were inserted into the incisions to discourage accummulation of blood in the wound, these drains are removed on the first postoperative day. Skin stitches are usually removed on the third to fifth postoperative day, and the healing wound may be supported with skin tapes for a while.

Removal of the elastic bands and wires from the teeth is a time of considerable anticipation for the patient. The exact time for this depends on the type of surgery performed and on other factors that may influence the rate of healing. Intermaxillary fixation usually lasts for six to eight weeks. Afterward, the jaws may be somewhat stiff. If necessary, the surgeon prescribes excercises that gradually increase their mobility and strength. The transition from a liquid diet to solids that are difficult to chew should be spread over several days. In some instances, physical therapy may help the return of normal function.

After the elastics and wires are removed, the surgeon carefully checks for evidence of incomplete bony healing. If present, intermaxillary fixation must be reinstituted for two to three weeks.

Complications of Orthognathic Surgery

In spite of the magnitude of orthognathic surgery, serious complications are unusual. However, excessive swelling in the early postoperative period may interfere with breathing and necessitate support of the airway. This complication, however, is extremely rare. The problem of nausea and vomiting has already been discussed.

Bleeding rarely occurs during the postoperative period, but if there is severe bleeding, a second operation may be needed for control. Accumulation of blood beneath the skin surface (hematoma) may predispose to swelling and infection and thus may require draining. Small rubber drains are frequently placed in the wounds to minimize the chances of hematoma.

Injury to the nerve that supplies the lower teeth and lips may produce lip numbness that is usually temporary but can be permanent. Injury to this nerve is more common in procedures that are performed on the tooth-bearing portion of the mandible than in those performed in the ramus (see preceding description). Injury to teeth is also less common in operations on the ramus.

Injury to the branch of the facial nerve responsible for movement of the lower lip may occur during procedures performed through skin incisions. Injury produces weakness of the lower lip that may be temporary or permanent. As the surgeon is aware of the position of this nerve and seeks to avoid it, injury is uncommon.

Because of the extensive blood supply of the head, infection following orthognathic surgery is unusual. If the healing bone becomes infected, however, the consequences can be devastating. Bone infection (*osteomyelitis*) is frequently difficult to control. It requires long periods of intensive antibiotic treatment coupled with surgical removal of diseased bone and can result in the failure of the bone fragments to heal (nonunion). If this occurs, a second operation may be required. Many surgeons routinely administer antibiotics just prior to and for several days after surgery to minimize the chances of infection.

Bony healing may fail for other reasons, such as inadequate immobilization of the fracture line, but this is extremely unusual. Superficial infection of the skin incision occasionally occurs, but is easily controlled with antibiotics or drainage.

On occasion the skin incision may fail to heal as expected and produce a noticeable scar. If this scar is objectionable, it may be minimized by scar revision (see chapter 7). Some people tend to form hypertrophic scars or keloids and those with a past history of this problem are carefully counselled preoperatively about this possibility.

Inadequate correction or a tendency toward recurrence of the jaw deformity occasionally follows orthognathic surgery. In many such cases orthodontic treatment may be beneficial, but in others a second operation may be required. If regression or development of an inability to completely close the front teeth is suspected during the first few days after the dental elastics and wires are removed, intermaxillary fixation is reinstituted.

Although these potential complications may seem formidable to the candidate for orthognathic surgery, it should be stressed that the diagnostic methods and surgical techniques currently in use result in an uneventful postoperative course for most patients. The rules of modern surgical practice dictate that, in spite of this, all patients must be counselled about possible complications before surgery. Although orthognathic surgery involves a more rigorous course than other forms of cosmetic surgery, the benefits in terms of improved appearance and function of the jaws and teeth far outweigh the hazards. Indeed, most people who have undergone this surgery are satisfied and say that they would do it again if necessary.

17

Otoplasty–Correction of Prominent Ears

Prominence of the ears because of excessive protrusion from the head (figs. 1 and 2) is relatively common. In contrast to other cosmetic facial deformities, which usually do not become apparent until later in life, prominence of the ears exists at birth. This condition appears to be hereditary, as it is more common in children of parents with protruding ears.

As prominent ears are present during the formative years of childhood, this condition may have considerable psychological impact on the developing personality and self-image. Although most children adjust to this problem, the name-calling and ridicule to which they are frequently subjected may result in considerable self-consciousness and anxiety. Young children are extremely perceptive of differences in appearance, and, as they are relatively uninhibited in their social interactions, such differences are freely pointed out. Many parents become aware of this potential problem and seek surgical correction by the *otoplasty* operation (*oto*—ear; *plasty*—repair or correction).

Anatomy of the Ear
Although there is considerable individual variation in the

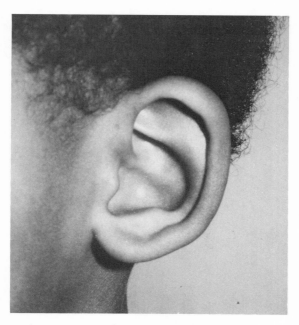

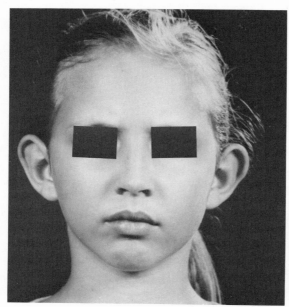

*Fig. 1 and 2.
Prominent
ears produced by
(a) deficiency of
antihelical fold,
(b) excessive
depth of the
conchal bowl,
(c) prominence
of the lobule.*

size and shape of the ear, all normal ears share certain anatomical features.

The skeleton of the ear—also called the *auricle* or *pinna*—consists of cartilage that exhibits multiple folds and convolutions. The overlying skin is relatively thin and adheres tightly to this skeleton, highlighting the convolutions of the cartilaginous skeleton (fig. 3). The ear lobe or *lobule* is suspended from the skeleton and consists of skin and underlying fat.

The average ear extends from the level of the eyebrow to the base of the nose and projects from the head at an angle of 15 to 30 degrees. This angle of projection is the major factor in prominence of the ears, a projection of more than 30 degrees producing such an appearance. The ears are usually slightly more prominent in men than in women.

Causes of Prominent Ears

Prominence of the ear is a consequence of altered development of the cartilaginous framework of the embryo. As noted, this development is genetically controlled. The mode of inheritance, however, is complicated and involves many genes. Other factors that operate during early fetal development may conceivably alter hereditary predisposition. Because of such factors, which may modify the expression (or penetrance) of genetic traits, the exact chance of children of an affected parent inheriting prominent ears cannot be predicted in each case. In general, however, the chances increase with the severity of the abnormality and are significantly greater if both parents have this problem.

Protrusion of the ear is occasionally caused by injury, or by surgical incisions made behind the auricle.

Anatomy of the Prominent Ear

Three basic anatomic abnormalities are responsible for the prominent ear. In most cases, the *antihelical fold* (fig. 3) is deficient, making the outer edge of the auricle project even further from the head. In many prominent ears, the depth of the *conchal bowl* (fig. 3) is excessive. The third contributing factor is protrusion of the ear lobe, or lobule. These features

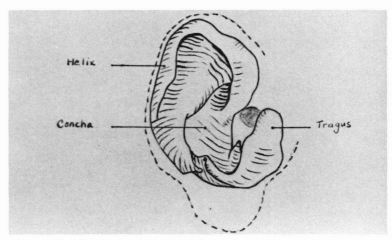

Fig. 3. Cartilaginous skeleton of the ear.

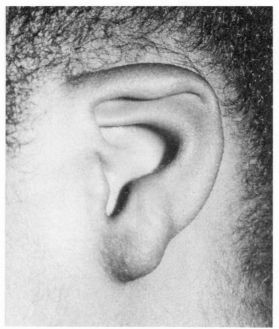

Fig. 4. "Lop ear."

are present in varying combinations in each individual case of prominent ears.

Occasionally a person has some other kind of deformity of the ear. Examples are the "lop ear," in which the upper part of the auricle is folded down (fig. 4) and the "satyr ear," in which the upper aspect of the pinna is pointed. In rare instances, more severe malformations of the ear, such as total absence of the auricle, occur. As such deformities are outside normal variation, they do not fall into the realm of cosmetic surgery as defined in chapter 1 and will not be discussed.

Historical Considerations

In addition to suffering ridicule and derision, before the twentieth century people with excessively prominent ears were in danger of being ostracized. Some scholars of those times associated deformities of the auricles with lack of intelligence, insanity, and criminal behavior. Critical scientific evaluation of those concepts, of course, has shown them to be invalid. These views were slow to disappear, however, and were mentioned in textbooks published as late as 1937.

Parents of children with prominent ears have long attempted to keep them from protruding by doing such things as taping the ears to the head during infancy. Such attempts, however, are of no proven benefit in altering the growth pattern.

Although the first otoplasty was performed in 1845, the procedure was not really accepted until 1910 when an American surgeon recognized the specific anatomic basis for protrusion of the ear and devised a procedure for correcting it. Since that time, many modifications and refinements of this operation have been introduced, and the contemporary cosmetic facial surgeon is, in most cases, able to realize the ultimate goal of otoplasty—production of an ear that looks natural, while avoiding the stigma of the "operated-on" look.

Selection of Candidates for Otoplasty

Candidates for otoplasty are carefully interviewed and examined. The causes of prominence of the ear are determined, and the general health of the patient is evaluated. Assessment of individual healing factors is important, as occasionally a patient develops unsightly scars on the back of the ear after otoplasty (see Complications of Otoplasty). Such a reaction occurs most often in dark-skinned people (see chapter 7).

As in all other cosmetic procedures, the motivation and expectations of the patient and parents are important factors. The motives for this procedure are usually obvious, but it must be realized that severe emotional or social problems will not be eliminated by surgery alone.

The expectations of patients and parents must be realistic. The goal of otoplasty is improvement in the appearance of the ears, not absolute symmetry and perfection. Most people's ears are not perfectly symmetrical. They vary in size and extent of protrusion. This is stressed during the surgeon's evaluation in an effort to avoid misunderstandings that may arise during the postoperative period.

Patients and parents must understand ear prominence occasionally recurs several weeks or months after otoplasty. Many contemporary techniques involve the use of sutures to maintain the ear in the position desired before the maturation of fibrous tissue that ultimately assumes this role. As in any mechanical system, sutures may fail and require replacement.

Age is an important factor in selecting candidates for otoplasty. The ideal age for this operation is five or six—i.e., just before the child's entry into kindergarten or elementary school. This is the period of greatest potential emotional trauma, and, by this time, the auricular cartilage is mature enough to withstand surgery. Surgery for girls is sometimes postponed until they are eight or nine, as protruding ears can frequently be camouflaged with hair. At this age, surgery can frequently be performed under local anesthesia.

Otoplasty is also performed on adults. The strength and resilience of the cartilage of this age group causes a slightly higher incidence of recurrence, particularly if sutures are used.

Preparation for Otoplasty

After accepting a candidate for otoplasty, the surgeon discusses important details of the surgical procedure and postoperative period, including his expectations concerning the patient's conduct during the critical postoperative healing period.

The location and extent of scars resulting from surgery are discussed, and the process of healing and scar maturation are described. The possibility of excessive scarring is mentioned (see Complications of Otoplasty), and other possible complications of the operation are reviewed.

Medical photographs are taken and discussed with the patient or parents. Particular emphasis is placed on associated defects and asymmetries that may have gone unnoticed and that may not be corrected by the otoplasty.

An informed consent agreement giving the surgeon permission to perform the operation is signed. Fees for otoplasty, as with other cosmetic procedures, are usually paid in advance (see chapter 1) and a member of the surgeon's office staff will make the appropriate arrangements.

Final Preparations for Otoplasty

The patient is instructed to avoid aspirin and other medications that may interfere with blood clotting for at least one week before surgery. He may be told to wash the face and shampoo with an antiseptic soap for several days before surgery to reduce the chance of postoperative infection. It is usually unnecessary to shave or clip the hair before surgery.

Hospital Admission

Most otoplasties performed on children are done in a hospital operating room, although operations on older children and adults are sometimes performed in outpatient facilities or office operating rooms. If surgery is scheduled in a hospital, the patient is usually admitted the evening before surgery for preoperative examination and laboratory tests. If surgery is to be performed in an outpatient facility, the patient is told to avoid solid food for six to eight hours before the operation to minimize the chance of vomiting.

Anesthesia for Otoplasty

Otoplasty is performed under both local and general anesthesia (see chapter 6). General anesthesia is almost always used for young children, while local anesthesia with sedation is used for older children and most adults. Sedatives are administered before the patient arrives in the operating room, and an intravenous infusion is started through which supplemental sedation can be given if necessary.

The Otoplasty Operation

The operative field is cleansed with antiseptic solution, and sterile drapes are positioned to prevent contamination of the area. The incision, made on the posterior surface of the auricle, consists of excising an ellipse of skin and subcutaneous tissue (fig. 5). The skin is then dissected from the posterior surface of the cartilaginous skeleton to allow its modification. A variety of procedures can be used to reshape the cartilage,

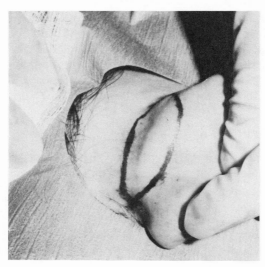

Fig. 5. Incision for otoplasty.

and the particular technique selected depends on the training and experience of the surgeon as well as on the type and extent of the abnormality that requires correction. Most techniques combine various modifications of cartilage incision or removal and use of sutures to manipulate the cartilage into the shape desired. Skin excision is frequently used to place the ear lobule in a satisfactory position.

The skin edges are then closed with sutures, and a sterile dressing is applied to the ear (fig. 6). The ear is protected from compression by soft cotton pads soaked in glycerin or mineral oil to help them conform to the convolutions of the auricle.

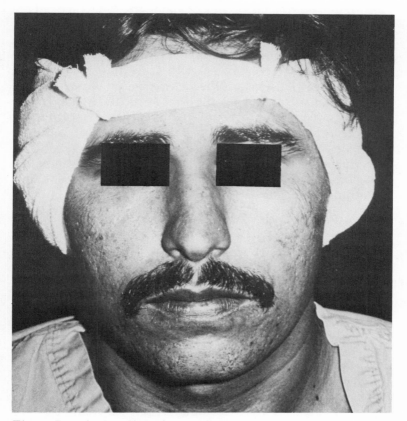

Fig. 6. Dressing applied after otoplasty.

Postoperative Care

The patient frequently experiences throbbing pain of moderate intensity in the first twenty-four hours after otoplasty. Bed rest and elevation of the head minimize this discomfort, and pain-relieving medications are prescribed as needed.

The dressing is removed the day after the operation and the ears carefully examined for signs of bleeding or accumulation of blood beneath the skin surface (hematoma). If a hematoma is found, it is promptly drained. At this time the ears are considerably swollen, discolored, and tender. The dressing is reapplied and left in place for four to seven days unless the patient complains of increasing pain. This symptom suggests development of a hematoma or infection and the ears should be inspected.

Although most of the discoloration has disappeared when the dressing is removed, the ear will remain tender and somewhat swollen for several weeks. In order to protect it from injury during this phase of the healing period, a tennis or ski headband is worn. During the first week the band is worn constantly. For about three weeks thereafter, it is worn while sleeping or playing. Injury during this period causes considerable pain and may predispose to bleeding or infection.

Sutures are removed five to seven days after the operation (figs. 7 and 8). Some surgeons use absorbable stitches that do not require removal.

Complications of Otoplasty

Significant complications rarely occur after otoplasty. The most common postoperative problems relate to bleeding. Frank hemorrhage, requiring reopening of the incision for control of the bleeding, is unusual. More frequent is accumulation of blood beneath the skin surface (hematoma). If these hematomas are not removed, they may result in cartilage damage and predispose to infection. Small hematomas can frequently be removed with a needle; larger collections may require reopening the wound or making an incision over their surface.

Infection rarely follows otoplasty, but its occurrence can be devastating if it spreads into the cartilage. For this reason,

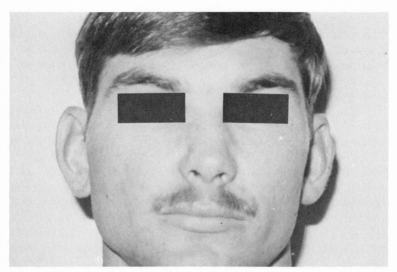

Fig. 7. Prominent ears of patient before correction surgery.

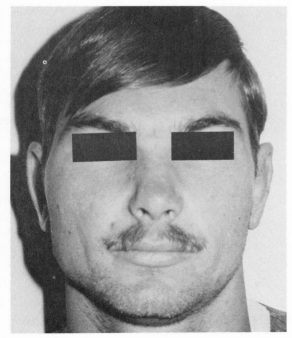

Fig. 8. The patient after otoplasty.

the ear is carefully inspected any time the patient complains of increasing pain in the early postoperative period. Redness of the ear, particularly around the incision, and low-grade fever are the other common signs of infection. Prompt administration of antibiotics and draining of localized areas of pus generally resolves infection.

Formation of excessive scar tissue around the incision occasionally follows otoplasty. The exact reasons for this reaction are obscure, but such hypertrophic scarring is more common in dark-skinned people. In many cases these scars gradually mature spontaneously. In others, injection of cortisone-like agents into the scar causes satisfactory resolution. Occasionally excision of the scar is required to control this reaction.

The possibility of recurrence of protrusion is carefully discussed with the patient preoperatively. Recurrence is most common when sutures are used to correct the deformity but may also occur in cases of cartilage incisions and removal. In such cases, a second operation is recommended to replace the ear in the desired position.

Overcorrection of prominent ears can also result in a "plastered down" appearance. Most patients are pleased with the surgical results anyhow and do not want to undergo a revision.

18

Adjuncts to the Face-Lift Operation

While the face-lift operation is effective in reducing signs of facial aging, this procedure alone cannot eliminate all the characteristics of the aging face. The face-lift, of course, is most effective in eliminating sagging, redundant skin around the jowls and upper neck.

Deep furrows in the forehead are not corrected by this procedure, and, although deep creases that extend from the base of the nose to the corner of the mouth, *nasolabial folds* (fig. 1), may receive some benefit from the standard face-lift, other procedures are required for more significant improvement. Deep vertical frown lines and the transverse crease often present at the root of the nose (horizontal frown line) also require ancillary measures.

The face-lift operation does not eliminate fine wrinkling. Such wrinkling is often improved by chemosurgery (see chapter 19) or dermabrasion (see chapter 20). Correction of the double chin and the firm bridlelike bands that often form in the front of the neck is not accomplished by the standard face-lift operation either. Methods of correcting these problems are discussed in chapters 15 and 23.

Redundancy and puffiness of the eyelid skin is not affected by the face-lift procedure. It requires the blepharoplasty operation (see chapter 12). While some improvement of the

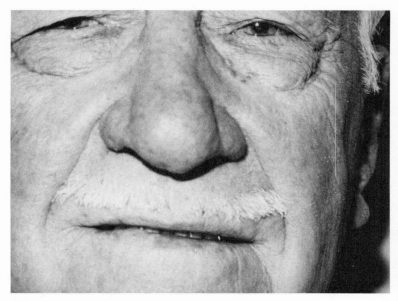

Fig. 1. Deep nasolabial folds.

sagging eyebrow may follow a face-lift, marked degrees of sagging can be corrected only by a brow lift (see chapter 13). Drooping of the nasal tip, which often occurs with aging, is not affected by face-lift surgery.

Contrary to popular opinion, the face-lift operation cannot improve the quality and texture of facial skin. Thin, poorly hydrated, leathery skin can not be rejuvenated into the smooth, resilient skin of youth by any surgical technique currently available.

Horizontal Forehead Wrinkles

The deep, horizontal creases in the forehead are among the first facial wrinkles to develop. Unlike other deep wrinkles that occur during aging, the horizontal forehead wrinkles occur largely as a result of activity of the underlying muscle (the *frontalis*—see chapter 9), rather than as a result of sagging and redundancy of aging skin. As a consequence, although these creases may be improved by surgical tightening of the forehead, this improvement will tend to be short-lived unless this muscle is rendered inactive. This can be done by partial removal of the muscle or by severing the nerve supply to the muscle during the operation. Although denervation may be very successful in accomplishing this goal, the resulting lack of forehead animation often appears unnatural. Also, motion of the eyebrows, frequently an important element of facial expression, is usually impaired by this procedure. In many cases, the eyebrows gradually sag after this procedure, resulting in a second deformity that requires correction.

The forehead lift is usually performed as an extension of the face-lift procedure but may be performed as a separate operation. The standard face-lift incisions continue above the ear to meet in the center of the scalp one to two inches behind the hairline (fig. 2). The forehead skin and attached frontalis muscle are elevated from the scalp to the level of the eyebrows. A portion of the frontalis muscle is usually removed at this time, and if the surgeon plans to injure the nerve

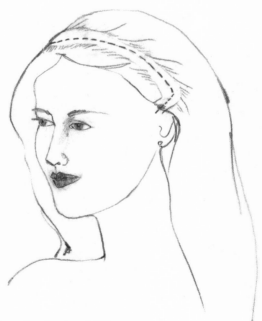

Fig. 2. Incisions for forehead lift.

supplying this muscle, it is identified. The forehead skin is then stretched into its proper position, excess skin removed, and the incision closed with sutures (figs. 3 and 4).

In addition to improving forehead wrinkles, this procedure tends to elevate the eyebrows, recreating the arching

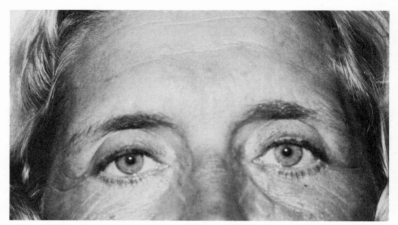

Fig. 3. Horizontal forehead wrinkles before surgery.

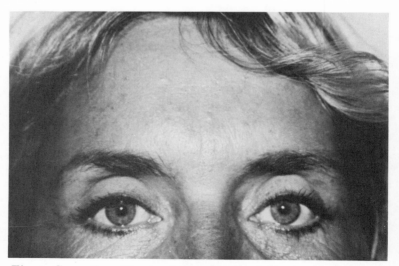

Fig. 4. Correction of horizontal forehead wrinkles by the forehead lift. Brows are also elevated by this procedure.

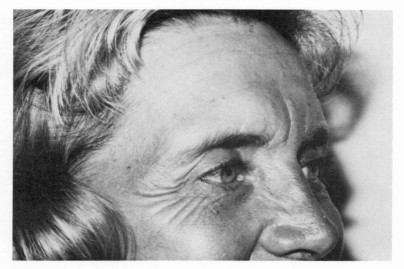

Fig. 5. Vertical frown lines before surgery.

sweep of youth. Many surgeons feel, however, that a more effective, longer-lasting brow lift is provided by incisions closer to the brow (see chapter 13).

Vertical and transverse nasal frown lines can also be corrected during the forehead lift by resection of the muscles that cause these wrinkles (figs. 5 and 6).

An absolute prerequisite for this operation is a satisfactory complement of forehead hair, which, of course, will be needed to camouflage the surgical scar. The forehead lift tends to elevate the frontal hairline and, in the case of people with abnormally high foreheads, the incision may be placed at the junction of the forehead and hairline. The scar is usually minimal and easily hidden by proper hairstyling.

Complications of the Forehead Lift

Complications after the forehead lift are similar to those that may follow face-lift surgery; namely, bleeding, accumulation of blood under the healing skin (hematoma), wound infection, and hair loss. A detailed discussion of these problems is found in chapter 11. Injury to nerves affecting the

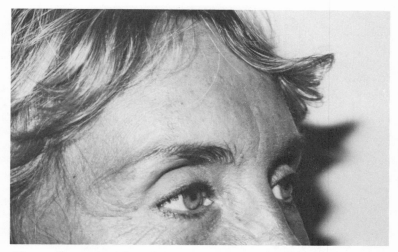

Fig. 6. Correction of vertical frown lines by the forehead lift.

sense of pain, touch, and temperature may result in numbness of the forehead. If such injury occurs, numbness is usually transient, as the injured nerve fibers regenerate.

Alternate Ways to Eliminate Forehead Creases

Some surgeons advocate direct excision of deep forehead wrinkles. After maturation the scars are relatively inconspicuous as they lie in the direction of natural forehead creases.

Dermabrasion (see chapter 20) and chemosurgery (see chapter 19) are sometimes beneficial in treating fine, superficial forehead wrinkles, but these techniques are disappointing when used on people with deep furrows.

Application of low voltage electrical current to the subcutaneous tissues under the creases is occasionally used to improve forehead creases. The object is to induce scarring beneath the creases, thus diminishing their depth.

A recently described treatment for forehead wrinkles consists of threading multiple fine sutures beneath the furrows. The suture material placed couples with the scar tissue that forms around these sutures and serves to fill in the depression.

Further studies are needed to properly evaluate this method of treating forehead wrinkles.

The procedure selected for treatment of the aging forehead depends on the extent and depth of wrinkling as well as the training and experience of the surgeon. Regardless of the method, recurrence of wrinkling may occur if the patient continues excessive use of the forehead muscles of expression. Counselling and retraining of habit patterns are essential for rejuvenation of the forehead.

Treatment of Vertical Frown Lines

These wrinkles also tend to develop at a relatively early age and result from the activity of the underlying corrugator supercilii muscles. Such wrinkles can be caused by constant squinting because of exposure to bright sunlight or poor vision. Frequent contraction of these muscles is a fundamental component of some people's facial expression, imparting an angry or concerned look.

Mild vertical frown lines can be treated by injections of small amounts of medical grade liquid silicone. Some surgeons advocate freeing the furrows from the underlying subcutaneous tissue through a small incision at the inner corner of the eyebrow. The corrugator muscles are then removed through this incision and the furrows are maintained in an elevated position with sutures for two to three days. Scar tissue forms under the wrinkles and tends to maintain elevation after suture removal.

Deep furrows are frequently treated by direct excision and skin closure; i.e., the wrinkle is treated as if it were a scar (see chapter 7). During this procedure, the corrugator supercilii muscles that cause the wrinkles may be excised. These muscles may also be excised in conjunction with the forehead lift or the eyebrow lift (see chapter 13).

Treatment of the Horizontal Frown Lines

In some people, frequent contraction of the *procerus muscle* (see chapter 9) produces a transverse crease at the root of the nose. Most such wrinkles can be effectively obliterated by silicone injections. Many surgeons, however, prefer to eliminate objectionable wrinkling by directly excising deep creases with or without removal of the underlying procerus muscle.

Treatment of the Deep Nasolabial Fold

Many people who request face-lift surgery are disappointed to learn that deep creases extending from the base of the nose toward the upper lips may not be dramatically improved by this operation. Ancillary procedures to improve the nasolabial folds may be recommended to these patients.

The most direct approach to this problem is excision of the redundant skin responsible for these folds—a technique called *nasolabioplasty* (fig. 7). The resulting scar is generally inconspicuous after maturation, as it resembles the natural nasolabial crease. Before maturation, the scar is often somewhat swollen and red, necessitating camouflage with cosmetics. Superficial infections of the healing wound may be a problem for patients with a thick, greasy skin. Frequent cleansing and use of appropriate antibiotics, however, helps control of such infection. Because of the necessity of incisions on exposed parts of the face, this procedure is not commonly used.

Deep nasolabial grooves may also be treated with injections of liquid silicone. Although such injections rarely completely

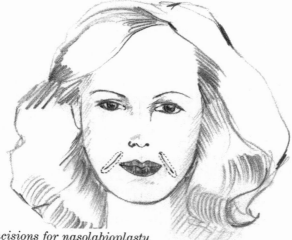

Fig. 7. Incisions for nasolabioplasty.

obliterate these furrows, significant improvement is often obtained. As noted, use of liquid silicone in cosmetic facial surgery is still being investigated, and thus liquid silicone is available to only a few cosmetic facial surgeons.

An older method for improving deep nasolabial folds is *linear eversion.* A small incision is made in the depths of the crease and a small knife or scissors inserted beneath the skin. The skin attachments to the subcutaneous tissue beneath the fold are severed and the skin adjacent to the fold is pulled into a ridge with sutures placed at frequent intervals. The goal is to induce scarring beneath the fold that results in its obliteration. A variant of this technique involves application of a low intensity electrical current to the subcutaneous tissue beneath the crease by means of a small needle placed through the skin. This current produces additional subcutaneous scarring.

Another method of treating the deep nasolabial fold involves placing fat grafts or artificial implants beneath the fold in an effort to fill in the depression with the implant and associated subcutaneous scarring. This method is relatively new and requires additional evaluation.

The Nose Lift

In addition to altering facial appearance, the gradual drooping of the nasal tip that accompanies aging can produce breathing difficulty. Many older people notice that elevating the tip with the fingers and restoring the normal patterns of air flow through the nose results in a dramatic relief of nasal obstruction (see chapter 14).

A modification of the rhinoplasty (see chapter 14) is often helpful in rejuvenating the nose's appearance and improving its function. This operation, sometimes called the "nose lift," consists of elevating the tip and supporting it in this position. In many cases, a small hump visible on profile, which became apparent as the tip gradually descended, will disappear after tip elevation. In other cases the small hump can be conservatively removed without requiring the controlled fractures of the nasal bones performed in the complete rhinoplasty. The results of the nose lift operation are frequently dramatic and do much to complement other procedures of facial rejuvenation.

19

Chemical Peel of the Face

The chemical peel—a form of chemosurgery—is a valuable technique for rejuvenating the aging face. It is an effective way to restore youthful vitality to facial skin with multiple fine wrinkles. As discussed in chapter 11, these wrinkles are not affected by the face-lift operation. The chemical peel, on the other hand, does not improve the general sagging and redundancy of the skin of the face and neck as does the face-lift operation. Thus, in many cases, the face-lift and chemical peel are complementary procedures.

The chemical peel is also useful in treating areas of abnormal pigmentation such as occurs on the upper lip and cheeks in association with pregnancy or the use of oral contraceptives.

History of Chemical Face-Peeling

Although the chemical peel has only gained approval as an accepted surgical technique since the early 1960's, this method has been used for many years. In the past, nonmedical operators of "beauty clinics" have applied chemical substances to various parts of the body in an attempt to rejuvenate the skin. Although the results were satisfactory in many cases, the complication rate was high and served to place such methods in disrepute. Cosmetic surgeons, however, became interested in chemosurgery and with careful modification and refinement of the chemical formula and techniques of application, the chemical peel has proven safe for properly selected patients.

Many patients who are candidates for chemical peel benefit from treatment of the entire face. Others, however, only exhibit fine wrinkling in some areas of the face and require treatment of only these areas. The regions most often treated in this manner are the skin around the lips, to eliminate fine vertical wrinkles (fig. 1) and the eyelid skin, to reduce fine wrinkling and "crow's-feet."

Selection of Candidates
for Chemical Peel

As with all other cosmetic facial procedures, proper selection of candidates is extremely important to obtain maximum benefit. In general, fair-skinned people with multiple, fine, facial wrinkling are the best candidates. Chemical peeling almost always causes a permanent decrease in skin pigmentation. This decreased pigmentation is more noticeable

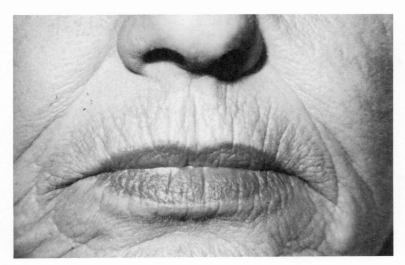

Fig. 1. Fine, deeply etched facial wrinkles amenable to chemosurgery.

in dark-complexioned people as the border between treated and untreated skin is often clearly evident. Most cosmetic facial surgeons are reluctant to accept these people for this reason.

The texture of the skin is another important factor in selection of candidates. The ideal candidate has relatively thin, moist skin. People with thick, oily skin are more apt to develop disturbances in pigmentation after this procedure.

The cosmetic facial surgeon must also assess the motivation and expectations of the candidate (see chapter 3). The postoperative course of chemical peel is perhaps more taxing than that of other cosmetic procedures, and the surgeon must be sure that the patient has enough emotional strength to weather it.

Candidates for chemical peel must understand that they must avoid exposure to direct sunlight for three to six months. They must also realize that as melanin production (see chapter 9) is permanently diminished by the peel, they may never again be able to get a dark tan. This prospect may be alarming to the person who wants fine facial wrinkles that may have largely been the result of years of sun worship removed, but this is the price of improvement by chemical peel.

The general physical condition of the prospective patient is assessed. For reasons discussed hereafter the surgeon is particularly interested in the condition of the liver and kidneys.

Preparation for Chemical Peel

After the candidate has been accepted for face peeling, the surgeon carefully counsels him about important details of the procedure and postoperative period. The expectations of the surgeon concerning the patient's conduct in the postoperative period are then discussed. These expectations center around proper skin care and strict avoidance of the sun.

Medical photographs are taken and reviewed with the patient so that the surgeon can carefully point out the areas that he proposes to improve as well as associated areas that will not be affected by the procedure. This is important in order to avoid disappointment in the postoperative period when the patient subjects his entire face to careful scrutiny.

The possible complications of face peeling are carefully explained and the patient is encouraged to ask questions about points he does not fully understand.

An informed consent agreement giving the surgeon permission to perform the procedure is signed.

Fees for the chemical peel are usually paid in advance (see chapter 1) and a member of the surgeon's office staff discusses this matter with the patient before final scheduling of the procedure.

The Chemical Peel

Chemical peel of the entire face is usually performed in the hospital, although treatment of small areas like the upper lip or eyelids may be performed on an outpatient basis. Hospitalization is preferred for the full face procedure because of the discomfort frequently experienced during the postoperative period.

The patient is instructed to wash his face with an antibacterial soap for several days before the procedure. Preoperative sedation is administered several hours before the procedure and an intravenous infusion is started through which he can be given additional sedation as required.

The active ingredient of the peeling solution is phenol, a substance that produces a superficial burn of the skin. Several other ingredients are added to promote even dispersion and penetration of phenol.

Before the chemical solution is applied, the face is carefully washed with surgical antiseptic and ether to remove all traces of oily material. The solution is applied to the skin with cotton-tipped applicator (fig. 2). The skin is gently stretched during application so that the solution will uniformly coat the skin and contact the bottom of each fine wrinkle. Application is continued into the hairline and eyebrows and just on to the red line of the lips in order to avoid visible lines of demarcation between treated and untreated skin. For the same reason, the application is continued to a point just below the border of the jaw. The neck skin is not peeled because a high incidence of scarring and abnormal pigmentation follows treatment of

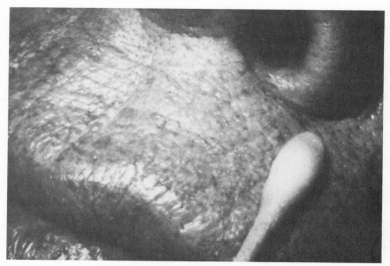

Fig. 2. Application of solution with cotton tipped applicator.

this area. Only a small amount of solution is applied to the eyelids as their skin is extremely thin.

A burning sensation is experienced for several seconds after the solution is applied. As phenol has local anesthetic properties, the burning sensation is quickly replaced by a relative numbness.

After the solution is applied, a mask of waterproof tape is applied to the skin. This mask prevents the phenol solution from evaporating and thus enhances its effect, producing a deeper and more uniform peel.

The Postoperative Period

Approximately one-half hour after the peel is completed, the patient begins to experience a burning sensation that gradually increases in intensity. Over the ensuing forty-eight hours this pain frequently requires narcotics for relief and this is a major reason for performing the procedure in a hospital.

The patient rests in bed with the head elevated, and, as chewing increases discomfort (as well as predisposing to premature loosening of the tape mask), a liquid diet taken by a straw is usually prescribed. For similar reasons, the patient is told to talk as little as possible. Iced compresses may be helpful in reducing pain during the first twenty-four hours.

On the second postpeel day, the tape mask is carefully removed and the raw area is covered with an antiseptic powder. The patient is heavily sedated at this time. The patient is usually discharged with instructions to apply the powder three times a day. Physical activity must be avoided while the face is powdered as perspiration may be troublesome.

Although the patient is frequently appalled at his appearance—in spite of the surgeon's preoperative warnings—pain has generally abated by now. There may be small blisters on the lips but these will disappear without treatment.

Application of bland ointment is begun twenty-four to forty-eight hours after the mask is removed in order to promote separation of the crust of powder and exudate from the face. On the next day, gentle washing of the face with bland soap and water is started to hasten crust separation.

The newly regenerating skin appears thin and delicate and has a reddish-pink color. After separation of the crust, no treatment is necessary other than frequent gentle washing and application of the bland ointment to help retain skin moisture. Ointments containing cortisonelike agents are sometimes prescribed. Cosmetics may usually be applied two weeks after the peel and are of benefit in masking the red color of the face.

Many patients complain of facial itching during this period. It may be extremely annoying and occasionally persists for several months. It is important not to scratch the face at this time as scarring could result. Medicine to diminish the itching can be provided if necessary.

Exposure to the sun must be carefully avoided for three to six months after chemical peel. If brief exposure is unavoidable, an effective sunscreen should be faithfully applied. Except for this precaution, patients may resume their usual method of skin care.

Complications of the Chemical Peel

Most complications following the chemical peel are related

to disturbances in skin pigmentation and are beyond the direct control of the surgeon. As these problems occur more frequently in people with dark complexions or thick, oily skin, such people are usually discouraged from undergoing this procedure.

A permanent decrease in skin pigmentation is always present after chemical peel and thus is not considered a complication. This bleaching effect results from a decrease in production of skin pigment (melanin) and as a result, the ability of the skin to produce a deep tan is decreased.

Some patients develop a noticeable line of demarcation at the junction of treated and untreated skin just below the jaw. This possibility is carefully discussed with patients preoperatively. If the line is objectionable, proper use of cosmetics can help conceal it.

Occasionally, areas of splotchy hyperpigmentation develop after a chemical peel. Again, this problem occurs most frequently in people with dark complexions, but may also occur in light-skinned patients after sun exposure. Repeeling of the face without application of a tape mask may be necessary to correct this abnormality. This second peel is delayed for at least three months after the initial procedure.

Pigmented facial blemishes present before the peel are frequently relatively darker after the procedure. As this is unavoidable, the only preventive measure is removal of objectionable blemishes before chemical peel.

Skin pores generally appear to be more prominent after a chemical peel. This is also unavoidable and candidates with large pores are carefully counselled regarding this effect prior to peeling. As pores are usually more prominent in people with thick, oily skin, this problem is more noticeable in such patients.

Pin-sized whiteheads called *milia* frequently occur after chemical peel. These areas are caused by temporary obstruction of small glands of the facial skin and, in most cases, can be satisfactorily treated by gentle washing. Some milia must be opened with a sharp needle.

Persistent redness of the facial skin sometimes occurs after a chemical peel. All patients develop redness after this procedure, but the rate of resolution varies. If redness is still

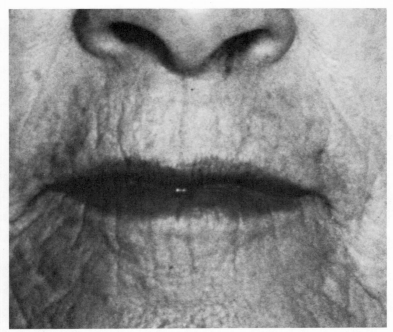

Fig. 3. Fine vertical wrinkles around the lips (before chemosurgery).

objectionable several weeks after the peel, application of creams or ointments containing cortisonelike agents may be helpful.

Significant infection of the skin rarely occurs after the chemical peel. Superficial bacterial contamination of the skin probably always occurs while the tape mask is in place, but it quickly resolves as the crust dries after antiseptic powder is applied.

Facial scarring after chemical peel is extremely unusual and occurs only if the peel extends too deeply or if the peel is followed by deep infection of the skin. As the chemical formula and the method of applying it to the skin are standardized, an excessively deep peel should rarely occur. If the surgeon suspects that a patient's skin is too delicate to tolerate the standard peel, he will not apply a tape mask after applying the solution. Full face peels are delayed for several weeks after a face-lift as excessive depth of the peel is more likely to occur if

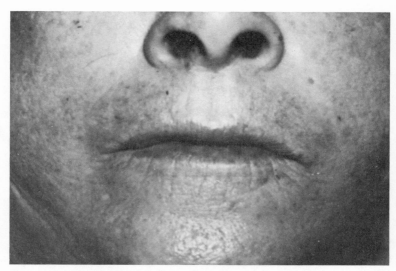

Fig. 4. Result of chemosurgery on upper lip.

these procedures are performed simultaneously. Chemical peel of the upper lip (figs. 3 and 4) is commonly performed in conjunction with the face-lift operation.

Mechanism of the Chemical Peel

Phenol, the active ingredient in the formula for chemical peel, produces a superficial burn of the skin. After healing, significant changes in the architecture of the skin can be observed under the microscope. The major change is a rearrangement of collagen fibers into a more orderly pattern. This microscopic change appears to be the factor responsible for elimination of fine wrinkling. Studies have shown that the changes in skin architecture are long lasting, correlating with the long duration of the improvement that frequently follows the chemical peel.

In spite of the complications that may follow chemical peel, it is the only method currently available for elimation of fine facial wrinkles. Most of the patients who undergo this procedure are extremely pleased by the effective and long-lasting facial rejuvenation obtained.

20

Dermabrasion

Dermabrasion is a method of mechanically removing the epidermal layer of the skin as well as the superficial part of the dermis in order to remove small, superficial skin irregularities and produce a smoother, more regular surface. If only the superficial layer of skin is removed, there are no scars. Deeper dermabrasion may result in scar formation, however, and dermabrasion in areas other than the face (removal of tattoos, etc.) almost always produces scarring.

Modern techniques of dermabrasion began in 1953 with development of the motor-driven abrader (fig. 1), which allowed precise, uniform, and rapid treatment of large areas of skin. Before this, some surgeons had used sandpaper to superficially abrade the skin surface. As this method was tedious and apt to produce nonuniform levels of abrasion, it was not widely used.

Uses of Dermabrasion

Perhaps the greatest value of facial dermabrasion is in its use for smoothing pitted facial scars produced by acne. The skin around these pitted areas is abraded to a lower level, diminishing the relative depth of the depressed areas. Although this technique has been widely publicized as a method

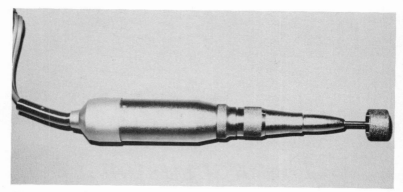

Fig. 1. Motor driven dermabrader.

of eradicating acne scars, the results are frequently disappointing, as they are directly proportional to the severity of the acne. Small, shallow scars can often be dramatically improved while larger, deeper pits receive little benefit. Again, as is true in all cosmetic facial surgery, improvement, not perfection, is a key consideration.

Dermabrasion is also useful in scar revision (see chapter 7). Six to eighteen months after surgery, small uneven areas between the scar and surrounding skin can be equalized by abrading the normal skin. The scar itself is not dermabraded as increased scarring may result.

This technique is also used for treatment of the vertical lines that appear around the lips during aging. Some surgeons have advocated dermabrasion for the "crow's-feet" appearing at the outer edge of the eye. This method has been largely superseded for treatment of fine wrinkles, however, by the chemical peel (see chapter 19), which produces a more satisfactory and lasting result. Superficial skin blemishes are occasionally removed by dermabrasion, allowing healing without visible scarring.

Dermabrasion is extremely useful in removing dirt and other contaminants from traumatic facial wounds. If such material is not removed, "tattoos" result as healing occurs around the imbedded debris. Removal after healing is extremely difficult. Dermabrasion is the most efficient, rapid, and effective method of cleaning such contaminated wounds.

Method of Dermabrasion

Dermabrasion is usually performed on an outpatient basis in the surgeon's office, but is occasionally performed under general anesthesia in a hospital operating room. After the skin is carefully cleansed with an antiseptic solution, the area to be treated is anesthetized. Anesthesia can be obtained by injection (see chapter 6) or by freezing the skin with a refrigerant. In addition to inducing anesthesia, freezing also makes the skin firmer, helping the surgeon obtain a uniform abrasion. Depressed areas are marked with dye to aid the surgeon in determining the proper level of abrasion of the surrounding skin.

The motor-driven dermabrader is then applied to the skin surface and the skin is abraded to the desired level. If a large area is to be treated, dermabrasion is performed in small units to insure a uniform skin removal.

Bleeding is controlled by pressure, and an occlusive gauze dressing applied. This gauze begins to spontaneously separate in three to five days and the patient is instructed to cover the healing area with an ointment. As the area heals, it appears intensely red, resembling a sunburn. This redness resolves over a period of time but in some cases is prolonged, particularly if the patient exposes himself to the sun.

Complications of Dermabrasion

Although dermabrasion is a relatively simple procedure, complications occasionally occur. Excessive prolonged redness of the skin, as noted, sometimes follows this procedure, but is unusual unless the patient suns himself or fails to protect his skin with an effective sunscreen for six to twelve months following treatment. Skin irritants, including those in ointment or cosmetics, are occasionally responsible for prolonged redness. This skin redness usually lasts for six to eight weeks.

Pin-sized white pustules called milia occur in about 50 percent of dermabrasion patients. These milia can generally be removed by washing with a wash cloth but occasionally require uncapping with a needle or surgical blade.

The most troublesome complications of dermabrasion are

pigmentation disturbances. Increased pigmentation is more common in dark-skinned people. Such patients must be thoroughly counselled about this possibility. Increased pigmentation is also more common after exposure to the sun. Pigmentation may be splotchy and it often takes months to years to completely resolve. On occasion, bleaching agents applied to the skin may help.

Areas of decreased pigmentation sometimes occur after dermabrasion, but are much less common than increased pigmentation. The reason for this is not known, but decreased pigmentation is more common after deep abrasion. If this condition does not resolve spontaneously, these areas may be camouflaged with cosmetics.

Scarring after dermabrasion of the face is uncommon but may occur if the level of abrasion has been too deep. Certain areas, including the neck and eyelids, are prone to scar formation. Consequently dermabrasion is not used in these regions. Scarring almost always occurs following dermabrasion of areas of the body other than the face. Patients with a tendency to form hypertrophic scars or keloids (see chapter 7) should not undergo facial dermabrasion.

Infection is an unusual complication of dermabrasion. If it occurs, it is usually superficial and is satisfactorily treated with cleansing and antibiotic ointments. If infection extends to the deeper layers, however, scarring may occur after destruction of the dermal tissue.

21

Correcting the Aging Neck

One of the most distressing features of aging is laxity of the skin of the neck that transforms the sleek, smooth profile of youth into a sagging redundant mass of flesh that at its most advanced is called the "turkey gobbler" neck. In many cases this sagging skin is accompanied by an accumulation of fat beneath the chin, producing a deformity known as the "double chin." Attempts to eliminate this double chin by dieting, exercise, or chin straps are uniformly unsuccessful. While correction of these problems is sometimes followed by the face-lift operation, often an extension or modification of this basic procedure is required. Many different approaches to surgical correction of the aging neck have been devised, but unfortunately none is universally applicable, and the surgical procedure must be tailored to the individual patient.

Anatomic Considerations

Ideally, the profile angle between the chin and neck approximates 90 degrees. The vertex of this angle is located over a small bone of the neck called the hyoid bone. In a pleasing profile the upper limb of this angle is approximately two-thirds of the length of the lower limb (fig. 1). A more obtuse angle is less pleasing to the eye, producing an appearance of

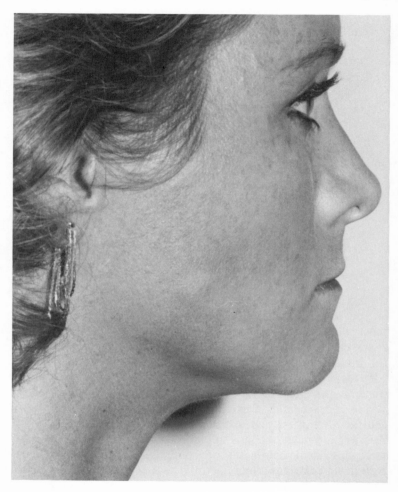

Fig. 1. Pleasing neck line.

webbing as compared to the sharp, well-defined 90-degree angle (fig. 2).

Webbing of the neck-chin angle may be the result of several factors. Sagging of lax neck skin and accumulation of fat beneath the chin are obvious causes. In some people, the hyoid bone develops in an abnormally low position. In such people the chin–neck angle is obtuse even in the absence of sagging

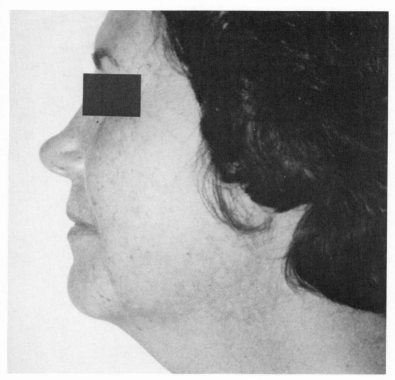

Fig. 2. Obtuse neck line with double chin.

skin. These people tend to form a double chin, secondary to fat deposition, at an early age. This tendency appears to be partly hereditary. Shortening of the horizontal limb of the chin–neck angle as a result of a relative deficiency or weakness of the chin (see chapter 15) may also contribute to an illusion of webbing (fig. 3).

Laxity of the superficial muscles of the neck may also contribute to the generalized sagging of the skin in this area. Of particular importance is the muscle of expression in the neck—the *platysma* (see chapter 9). In some people this muscle thickens, forming two bridlelike bands that project beneath the skin of the front of the neck. A hollow or depression between these bands increases their prominent appearance (fig. 4) producing the "stringy" neck.

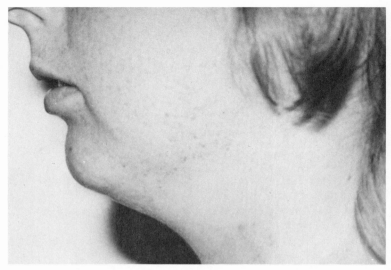

Fig. 3. "Chin weakness" accentuates illusion of webbing of neck.

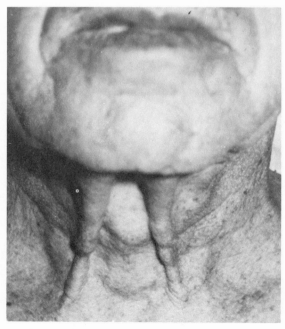

*Fig. 4.
Bridlelike
bands in neck
formed by
platysma muscle.*

Correcting the Aging Neck

There are several operations that attack the causes of the aging neck. The degree of skin laxity and the extent to which fat accumulation and muscle prominence contribute to the problem are the factors that determine which operation is selected. As sagging of the neck skin is almost always accompanied by laxity of the facial skin, these procedure are usually planned in conjunction with the face-lift.

Most surgeons initially approach the aging neck with modifications of the face-lift operation. The neck skin is widely undermined to allow it to be "lifted" maximally. The location and configuration of the part of the face-lift incision behind the ear and in the hairline may be modified to allow greater pull on sagging neck skin. Some surgeons believe that plication of the superficial neck muscles with stitches helps produce a more effective "neck lift."

If accumulation of fat beneath the chin or "bridling" of the platysma muscle accompanies relaxation of neck skin, these modifications of the face-lift operation will not produce satisfactory correction. Some surgeons remove this supplemental fat through a small incision under the chin (fig 5). The edges of the platysma muscle responsible for the bridled appearance can also be approached through this incision. Some surgeons prefer to suture these muscles together to eliminate this problem, while others feel that partial removal of the muscles yields better results. These procedures are often performed at the time of face-lift surgery. In some cases, however, the surgeon prefers to perform these corrections six to eight weeks after the face-lift. At this time, the extent to which the face-lift has improved the neck appearance will be evident and correction of the residual deformity can be planned accordingly.

In cases of marked redundancy of the neck skin that produce the "turkey gobbler" neck, more extensive corrections may be needed. Direct excision of skin by means of incisions in the neck may be necessary to achieve an optimum result. Incisions of various configurations have been advocated, and the type of incision employed is selected after careful evaluation of the individual patient. Unfortunately, these incisions produce visible scars, a fact which is carefully explained to

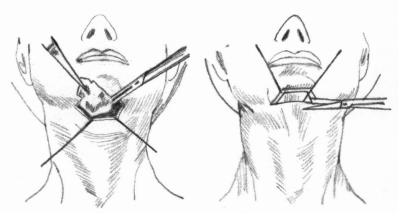

Fig. 5. Incision placed beneath chin for removal of fat producing double chin.

the patient before the operation. The scars vary from individual to individual as a result of differences in wound healing determined by factors discussed in chapter 7. These operations are almost always performed six to eight weeks after the face-lift as the skin tension in the neck that results from the face-lift would tend to widen the scars if both procedures were performed simultaneously.

Augmentation of a weak chin (see chapter 15) is a useful adjunct in improving the appearance of the neck. Lengthening the upper limb of the chin–neck angle by this method tends to enhance the appearance of this angle.

One important factor that limits the surgeon's ability to improve the appearance of the neck is the position of the hyoid bone. The position of this bone determines the vertex of the chin–neck angle. Low placement of the bone produces a more obtuse angle, and as the surgeon cannot change its position, correction of the chin–neck profile is limited.

Selection of Candidates for Surgery of the Aging Neck

As most patients undergo these procedures in conjunction with the face-lift, the important features of patient selection and preparation are similar to those described for face-lift surgery (see chapter 11). When examining the patient, the cosmetic surgeon assesses the relative contributions of skin, fat, and muscle in producing the signs of aging. The position of the hyoid bone is also noted for the reasons previously discussed.

If neck incisions are planned, the patient is carefully warned of the possibility of telltale scars. The processes of wound healing and scar maturation are also discussed.

As with face-lift surgery, the supplemental operations designed to correct the aging neck may be performed either in an outpatient surgical facility or a hospital operating room. Although most such operations are performed under local anesthesia, some surgeons use general anesthesia.

Complications in Correction of the Neck

If the aging neck is rejuvenated by a modification of the face-lift operation, the significant complications possible are

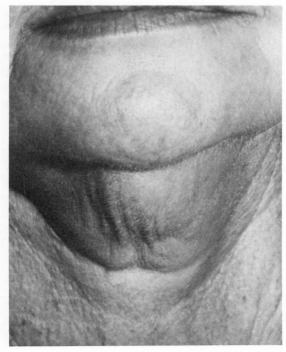

Fig. 6. Accumulation of fat in the neck, frontal view.

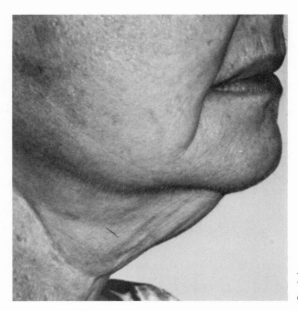

*Fig. 7. Side
view of this
condition.*

similar to those described in the discussion of that procedure
(see chapter 11). Attempts to stretch the sagging neck skin
tightly are probably associated with a higher frequency of scar
widening and skin loss than in the routine face-lift procedure.

One troublesome complication that may follow fat removal
through an incision under the chin is adherence of the incision to the underlying muscle. This produces a noticeable
depression. This problem is usually related to overzealous
excision of fat and can usually be prevented by leaving a
small amount of fat attached to the undersurface of the skin.

As scars normally result from operations that necessitate
neck incisions, they are not true complications of these procedures. The patient is always warned that these scars may
widen and become objectionable and this possibility must be
carefully weighed against the benefits expected from surgery.

Most patients, however, are willing to accept scars to obtain correction of double chins (figs. 6 and 7) and sagging
neck skin. If scars are troublesome to the patient, scar revision (chapter 7) may be helpful.

22

Hair Transplantation

Complete or nearly complete loss of scalp hair is a condition that ultimately affects 10 to 15 percent of the male population. Although some men have used baldness to enhance their images and further their careers, for most, adjustment to it is emotionally painful. This is evidenced by the sales of hairpieces and advertising of products that promise to preserve hair or stimulate its growth. Younger men may be particularly apprehensive and lose their self-confidence because of baldness.

Hair loss may also occur in women but it tends to be a diffuse thinning rather than the complete baldness on the forehead region and vertex characteristic of men.

Hair transplantation offers people a way to combat balding. Many misconceptions, however, surround this procedure. The results are limited, and miraculous transformations are seldom achieved. A full head of hair cannot be expected, as transplanted hair is always less dense than normal hair. Unfortunately, results are generally better for men with the least-advanced hair loss.

Male Pattern Baldness

By far the most common type of hair loss is male pattern

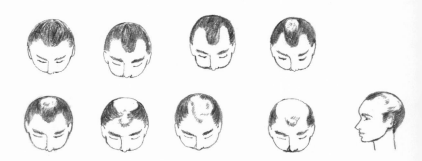

Fig. 1. Variations of male pattern baldness.

baldness, a condition that accounts for more than 95 percent of baldness in adults. This type of hair loss is called pattern baldness because it characteristically produces distinct patterns that show a predictable progression (fig. 1). The most common pattern begins as a recession of the outer part of the forehead hairline in a symmetrical triangular configuration (fig. 1). This leaves a peninsula of hair in the middle of the forehead. Such patterned hair loss starts casually in the late twenties or early thirties and progresses at a variable rate.

For many people with this type of pattern baldness, hair loss also occurs in the vertex. As hair loss in these areas continues, they become confluent leaving a characteristic rim of hair in the temples and back of the scalp.

Another pattern of baldness is characterized by gradual recession of the entire forehead hairline without preservation of a central peninsula, which continues toward the vertex without concomitant hair loss in the vertex.

Although the exact cause of male pattern baldness is unknown, a combination of three separate factors—male hormones (*androgens*), heredity, and aging—appear to be important in determining the extent of this condition.

The exact hereditary basis of male pattern baldness has not been determined. A common idea is that this condition is inherited through the mother on a set chromosome—the X-chromosome. A more probable theory, however, is that male pattern baldness is inherited through both mother and father on a nonsex chromosome. According to this hypothesis, levels of male hormones interact with this genetic information to ultimately determine baldness, explaining the infrequency of baldness in the female. As the age of onset of this form of pattern baldness varies considerably in different people, as does its progression and ultimate extent, this is undoubtedly an oversimplification. Many other hereditary and environmental factors probably interact to determine these variables.

The role of aging in balding is obvious. With increasing age, the areas of baldness extend and in many cases become confluent. Nearly 95 percent of men show some patterned hair loss by sixty-five. Five percent of men destined to have pattern baldness notice significant hair loss before they are twenty. In 1 to 2 percent of men, pattern baldness is severe by thirty.

Considerable racial differences exist in male pattern baldness. This condition tends to be more common and more marked in Caucasians. Blacks demonstrate a lesser incidence, and baldness is least common in Orientals.

Hair Loss in Adolescence

Diffuse thinning and recession of the forehead hairline occurs in approximately 95 percent of boys and 80 percent of girls during early adolescence. This hair loss is often a source of considerable anxiety to teenage boys, especially those with a family history of baldness, but it usually does not indicate the onset of pattern baldness. This characteristic also has a hereditary basis but is not necessarily inherited in association with pattern baldness. As noted previously, only about 5 percent of men who develop pattern baldness begin to do so before twenty.

Other Causes of Baldness

While most baldness is of the male pattern type, many other factors may be responsible for localized or diffuse temporary or partial hair loss. Disease of the scalp that produces scarring in or beneath the skin may permanently destroy hair follicles. Similarly, acute injury or chronic traumatic insults such as frequent pulling of the hair, or lying in one position, may damage the hair follicles. (Infants who sleep on their backs frequently have temporary hair loss over the back of the head.)

Exposure to radiation or certain toxic chemicals or medication used for treatment of cancer may be responsible for temporary or complete baldness.

Hair loss may also result from hormonal disorders caused by disease of the thyroid, pituitary, or adrenal glands as well as the ovaries. Some women experience a temporary hair loss during pregnancy or after childbirth.

Infection of the scalp by various fungi, bacteria, and viruses may also cause hair loss. Baldness can occur during severe generalized illnesses, too. The role of psychologic factors alone in causing hair loss is uncertain.

Contrary to popular opinion, there is no evidence to suggest that dandruff or other common disorders of the scalp significantly accelerate hair loss. Some dermatologists, however, advocate aggressive treatment on the grounds that slight acceleration of other causes of baldness may occur.

In some cases extensive evaluation, usually coordinated by a physician specializing in disorders of the skin (dermatology), is required to determine the exact cause of hair loss.

Characteristics of Scalp Hair

Hair originates from appendages of the epidermis called follicles located below the skin surface. The hair root, which develops inside the follicle, contains a matrix of living cells. Division of these cells is responsible for production of a protein material (*keratin*) that forms the hair shaft. Hair grows in a cyclic manner. The phase of continuous growth of scalp hair lasts several years, then slows for several weeks before entering a resting phase that lasts for several months. The average human scalp contains 100,000 to 140,000 hairs, all of which are in independent growth cycles; therefore, scalp hair grows continually. Only a small number of follicles are in a resting phase at any given time. A hair grows an average of 4 millimeters a day and lives an average of four years.

Hair color is determined by granules of melanin pigment present in the hair shaft. Darker hair, of course, has a higher concentration of pigment granules. When pigment production ceases, usually as a result of aging, the hair becomes gray. Dark hair tends to be coarser than blonde or red hair.

The shape of each individual hair shaft determines whether the hair is straight or curly. Straight hairs are circular, while curly hairs are oval shaped.

Baldness can occur as a result of losing hair shafts while the follicle continues to live or as a result of damage or death of the follicle itself. If the hair follicle continues to live, baldness is temporary; follicular death causes permanent baldness.

As noted, male pattern baldness is caused by the interaction of hereditary, aging, and hormonal factors. Hair follicles in the areas of baldness seem to be programmed to die at certain ages in the presence of a sufficient level of male hormones. The follicles in areas where hair growth continues do not respond to hormonal stimulation in this manner. This is the basis of hair transplant surgery. Hairs taken from areas where there is no baldness will continue to grow after they are transferred to bald areas because of this genetically determined behavior.

Selection of Candidates for Hair Transplantation

Although development of hair transplant procedures has given many balding men new hope for hair restoration, these procedures are not suitable for all people and so candidates must be carefully evaluated. As in most aspects of cosmetic surgery, improvement rather than perfection is the rule. In spite of popular notions, there are few miraculous transformations.

Of prime importance in selecting candidates is the extent of hair loss and the density of the remaining hair. This is because hair transplanted into bald areas must be obtained from areas that still have hair. In evaluating younger men whose pattern of baldness has not stabilized, the surgeon must attempt to predict the ultimate extent of hair loss and use hair from areas that will not become bald as the patient ages. As previously discussed, these follicles can be expected to survive indefinitely as they have not been genetically programmed to respond to male hormone levels by ceasing to grow, as have hair follicles in bald areas.

The best candidates for hair transplantation are those with moderate recession of the forehead hairline who merely desire some restoration of the hairline. Ideal candidates also have dark, coarse hair that is relatively dense in areas that have hair. Men with marked degrees of pattern baldness seldom obtain significant improvement from hair transplantation because the density of transplanted hair rarely approximates the natural density and suitable donor areas are limited.

The cause of hair loss is also important. Most hair transplantation procedures are performed because of male pattern baldness, but hair loss secondary to some of the factors discussed may also be treated in this way. The primary disorder, of course, must have been resolved and the scalp must be healthy enough to support the transplanted hair follicles.

The general health of the candidate is an important factor in selection. Patients with chronic disorders such as diabetes or high blood pressure may be unsuitable. Some surgeons refuse to perform this procedure on patients with cardiac histories.

As in all cosmetic surgery, psychological factors are important in selection of candidates (see chapter 3). Of particular concern are the motives and expectations of the patient. The motivation must be strong to endure the inconveniences of the multiple procedures required. The exceptations of the patient must be realistic. He should thoroughly understand the limitations of the procedure, especially the fact that transplanted hair is never as dense as normal hair. He must accept the fact that improvement, rather than perfection, is the goal.

Preoperative Instructions

Most hair transplant procedures are performed in an office operating room or other outpatient surgical facilities, and little preoperative preparation is needed. The patient is usually told to wash his hair daily with an antibacterial shampoo for several days before the procedure.

As bleeding may be a problem, patients should not take aspirin for at least one week before surgery. If other medications are being taken, the surgeon will determine whether or not they should be discontinued before the procedure.

The Hair Transplant Procedure

When the patient arrives in the office operating room, his scalp donor area and recipient sites are cleansed with surgical antiseptic. These areas are then clipped with small scissors. The clipped part of the donor area is hidden by adjacent hair after the procedure is completed.

Anesthetic solution is then injected into the scalp. This solution contains adrenalin, which constricts the small blood vessels of the scalp and reduces bleeding. Many surgeons perform the procedure with the patient sitting up to further reduce blood loss.

The operation itself consists of cutting small circular plugs (usually four millimeters in diameter) from the donor area and transplanting them into defects of similar size, which are created in the recipient area. These grafts consist of full thickness skin incorporating fifteen to twenty hair follicles (fig. 2). They are obtained with a specially designed skin

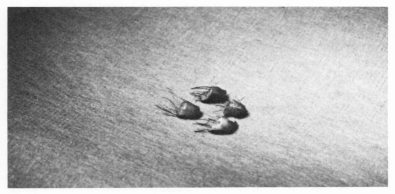

Fig. 2. Hair plugs for transplantation.

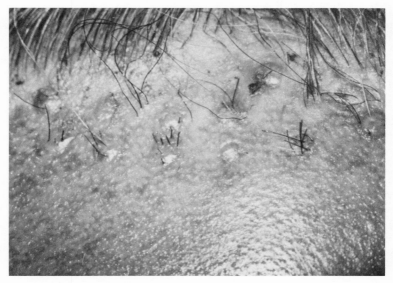

Fig. 3. Hair plugs in place.

punch. As these follicles have been programmed not to respond to male hormones, they will continue to produce hair in
the donor site (fig. 3). Many surgeons transplant 25 to 50
plugs per session but others, using newly developed power
driven punches, transplant 100 to 150 plugs per session. Typi-
cally, sessions are at two to three week intervals, although
transplantation in another area can be performed as early as
the following day. Six to twelve procedures are usually required for an optimal result.

An alternate method of creating a new frontal hair line is
transplantation of long, narrow strips of hair-bearing scalp.
This technique may allow a more rapid restoration of the
forehead hairline in properly selected patients. Some surgeons, however, report a higher incidence of graft failure
with this technique as compared to the punch graft method.

The Postoperative Period

After the hair transplant procedure is completed, a soft,
nonadherent dressing is applied to the donor and recipient

areas. A turbanlike bandage is applied next and left in place for twenty-four hours. After this dressing is removed, the grafted area is gently cleansed with hydrogen peroxide to remove small crusts that develop adjacent to the grafts. If necessary, the position of the plugs is adjusted at this time.

The graft site can be covered in a variety of ways during the early healing period. If there is enough adjacent hair, it can be combed over the treated area. Some surgeons allow use of hairpieces over the grafted area as early as the first day after surgery—as long as no adhesives or other attachments are applied to the graft sites. Others, however, recommend avoiding hairpieces for a week. Small dressings, covered with flesh-colored tape, can also be applied for camouflage.

The patient is told to avoid strenuous activity for five to seven days as perspiration may have an adverse effect on the healing grafts. Adjacent hair must be combed and brushed with care to avoid graft injury.

Gentle shampooing can begin on the fifth postoperative day. Careful attention to cleanliness is essential as crusts may form in the grafted area for ten to twenty days after the operation. These crusts may cause annoying itching, but the temptation to scratch must be resisted.

Pain following hair transplant surgery is generally minimal and can usually be controlled with mild analgesics. Aspirin is not recommended as it may predispose to bleeding.

In some patients swelling of the forehead area appears on the second or third postoperative day and lasts for five to six days. This swelling, which tends to be more frequent and severe when large numbers of grafts are inserted, may be accompanied by discoloration of the upper eyelids.

Results of Hair Transplantation

After a successful hair transplant, the grafted hair appears to grow for the first three to four weeks. This hair, however, soon falls out as the follicles enter the resting phase of the hair cycle. New hair growth begins ten to twelve weeks after the procedure. As hair grows at a maximum rate of four millimeters a day, significant hair growth does not become apparent for at least six months. The final results of hair transplantation cannot be realistically assessed for twelve to eighteen months postoperatively. Regardless of the degree of survival of the grafts, a full head of dense hair cannot be expected. This fact, coupled with the patience with which the final result must be awaited, are reasons that the candidate for hair transplantation must be carefully counselled before starting this lengthy series of procedures.

After the transplanted hair grows, it can be styled and dyed as desired.

Complications of Hair Transplantation

Serious complications from hair transplant surgery are extremely unusual, but if they occur, the final result may be compromised. The most devastating complication, of course, is failure of the grafts to grow hair. Unfortunately, such failure may not be obvious for several months after surgery. In many cases, nonfunctioning grafts can be replaced.

Some patients develop a persistent, irregular "cobble-stoned" appearance in grafted areas as a result of growth of the plugs at different areas. This appearance usually resolves in six to twelve months.

Occasionally grafted hair changes in texture and color, becoming more coarse, curly, and dark. In many instances, this change is beneficial as the hair appears denser in these areas.

Improper graft placement may create a forehead hairline that appears unnatural. As experience with hair transplantation has increased, most surgeons have become aware of the problems of attempting to reconstruct the hairline too far forward, and thus the incidence of this complication has markedly decreased.

Excessive scarring after hair transplantation can cause serious problems, compromising growth of hair and altering the scalp's appearance. Fortunately, this complication is unusual. The appearance usually gradually improves with time and after scar maturation it may be possible to perform additional grafting.

Superficial infection, manifested by redness and swelling around the grafted areas, is fairly common, but deep infection following hair transplantation is rare. If uncontrolled, infection may predispose to scarring, compromising the final result.

Mild oozing of blood from the graft site is common during the immediate postoperative period, but vigorous bleeding is unusual.

Alternatives to Hair Transplantation

Several alternatives are available to balding people who do not want to undergo hair transplantation.

HAIRPIECES

Perhaps the most common method of camouflaging a bald scalp is with a hairpiece or toupee. Many people, however, complain that these hairpieces do not look natural and worry that they may become displaced at inopportune times. Such vigorous activities as swimming and other forms of physical exercise that cause perspiration cannot be indulged in while wearing a hairpiece. Natural hair must be trimmed frequently so that it blends with the toupee. The hairpiece itself requires care and occasionally causes irritation and itching.

HAIR WEAVING

In this process tufts of artificial hair are woven into a person's residual hair. This artificial hair is relatively stable and it allows a person to do many things he could not do when wearing a conventional hairpiece. The woven hair, however, does loosen with time as the natural hair in which it is anchored grows. Generally it must be rewoven or tightened at intervals of two to ten months. Hair weaving is most effective when there are only small bald areas that must be covered. This technique is not usually satisfactory for advanced balding as there isn't enough hair available to anchor the hairpiece. It may be difficult to clean the scalp after hair weaving.

COSMETIC HAIR REPLACEMENT OR HAIR IMPLANTATION

This is a relatively new procedure in which artificial hair is attached to the scalp with a net of sutures or thin wires placed into the scalp by a physician. This forms a semipermanent hairpiece that does not require removal and allows a person to be active. The artificial hair is styled and can be combed, brushed, and shampooed almost as normal hair.

Several potential problems, however, are associated with this technique. The scalp sutures may irritate the skin, become infected, and require removal. Some people complain of a sensation of tightness in the scalp and may have frequent headaches. Because of these problems, frequent revisions of scalp sutures may be required during the period of adjustment. Natural hair may have to be frequently trimmed to make it blend with the artificial hair. Also, it may be difficult to keep the scalp clean beneath the hairpiece.

A continual parade of products advocated for preservation of hair or stimulation of hair growth from bald scalps are advertised in the media. These products include various tonics, moisturizers, shampoos, massage units and innumerable other devices. Various diets and vitamin supplements have also been advocated for treatment of baldness. While good scalp hygiene is certainly helpful in maintaining healthy hair, there is no evidence that any of these tonics or devices are of value in retarding or minimizing hair loss in male pattern baldness. In some patients whose baldness is secondary to other causes, medical treatment prescribed by a dermatologist may be of value in arresting hair loss or stimulating hair growth.

German investigators have recently discovered that a chemical agent used for treatment of cancer stimulates hair growth in men with pattern baldness. Such hair growth has been temporary and generally of low density. It should be emphasized that these investigations are preliminary. A lot more study will be needed to determine whether or not modifications of this technique will be valuable in treating baldness. Until that time, people who want to reverse their baldness should seek hair transplantation or the other reputable methods described in this chapter.

Future Trends in Hair Transplantation

SCALP FLAPS

A method of restoring hair by transferring large areas of hair-bearing scalp to bald areas has generated considerable interest among cosmetic surgeons. This transferred tissue, called a flap, differs from the conventional scalp grafts in that it remains attached to its original blood supply after transfer and so does not depend on the recipient area for nourishment. The hair follicles in the scalp flap do not shed their hair and so this method may produce "instant results." The flap donor site is closed with sutures and heals with a scar hidden by adjacent hair (figs. 4 and 5).

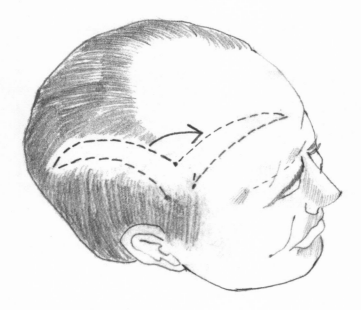

Fig. 4. Scalp flaps for hair.

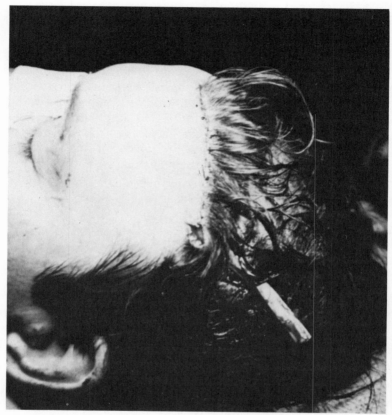

Fig. 5. Scalp flap immediately after transposition.

While this technique is new and not currently suitable for all balding people, it offers considerable promise. Further technical refinements will undoubtedly extend its usefulness (figs. 6 and 7).

HAIR BANKS

Transfer of hair from one person to another is currently limited by the problem of rejection by the body of skin and other tissues that are transplanted from another person. Experiments are being done in this area and perhaps some day the problem of rejection can be overcome, allowing formation of hair banks and extending the availability of hair for transplantation.

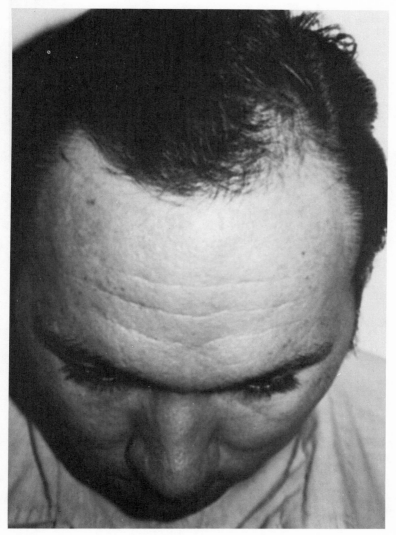

Fig. 6. Patient before transposition of scalp flaps.

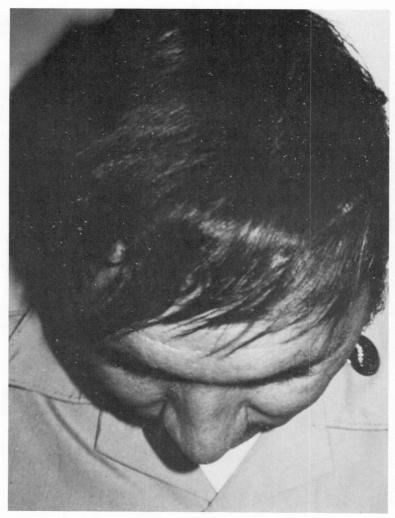

Fig. 7. After two scalp flaps have been transposed.

SCALP REDUCTION

A new addition to the armamentarium of the hair transplant surgeon is the technique of scalp reduction. A portion of bald scalp is removed, rather than transplanted with hair plugs. The edges of the resulting defect are loosened by separating them from their underlying attachments so that they can be sewn together, producing a fine linear scar. Scalp reduction is usually performed under local anesthesia and results in a substantial saving of hair plugs that can be used for producing increased hair density in the remaining areas of the transplanted scalp. Reduction can be performed before punch grafting or at any time between sessions of grafting.

23

Cosmetics and Hairstyling as Adjuncts to Facial Surgery

Appropriate use of makeup and intelligent selection of a hairstyle can make a positive contribution to facial appearance. Cosmetology and hairstyling are complex and dynamically changing areas. As facial surgeons are rarely expert in these subjects, this discussion will focus only on general concepts pertinent to use of cosmetics and hairstyling as adjuncts to surgery.

The Use of Cosmetics

In spite of the current emphasis on the "natural look," there are few women whose appearance cannot be enhanced by judicious use of cosmetics. Actually, the philosophy of the "natural look" is entirely consistent with the use of makeup to enhance and draw attention to attractive features. This approach is in direct contrast to the older concept of using makeup to cover or camouflage less desirable features—an approach that often resulted in an artificial look.

Although few facial surgeons are knowledgeable in the basic techniques of cosmetic use, most are impressed with the way appropriate makeup enhances surgical results. Many surgeons routinely suggest that their patients consult a cosmetologist or makeup artist postoperatively. Some women feel that such a consultation is unnecessary. After all, most of them have been using makeup regularly for many years and feel that their proficiency is more than adequate. It is important to realize, however, that the facial structure and appearance is altered by surgery, and the use of cosmetics should be altered accordingly to enhance and maximize the appearance. This is especially important after eyelid and face-lift surgery as preoperative makeup techniques were undoubtedly directed toward hiding wrinkles and sagging skin.

Consultation with a cosmetologist is valuable for several reasons. The selection and proper use of the large and often bewildering array of products available depends on an objective analysis of the individual face. In addition to providing objective analysis of facial proportion, features, balance, and skin texture, cosmetologists are familiar with new products and the philosophy and techniques of applying them. These new ideas and techniques are easily learned and incorporated into a person's own routine.

Ideally, makeup consultants should not be affiliated with any one brand of cosmetics but should be free to recommend products of several manufacturers. Most cosmetic surgeons can recommend such consultants.

Hairstyling as a Frame for the Face

In general, hair can be thought of as a frame for the face. Just as a frame should not draw attention from the picture it surrounds, an ideal hairstyle should complement, rather than distract from, the face.

Proper styling and shaping of the hair helps considerably to achieve a desirable facial balance, proportion, and symmetry. Subtle use of color, tint, and highlighting further enhances the appearance of the face.

As in cosmetology, philosophies of hairstyling have undergone considerable changes in the past several years. Older concepts held that proper hairstyle should be determined by the shape of the face. Thus square faces could be transformed into the more desirable oval shape by using long hair to cover a square jaw line, and high foreheads could be camouflaged by long bangs. Adhering to these principles often resulted in hairstyles that overwhelmed the face.

New concepts of styling hold that the shape and proportion of the hair itself, rather than the shape of the face, is the most important factor in achieving balance and compatibility with the face. Actually, the best philosophy probably lies between these extremes.

Realistically, the texture, thickness, and extent of natural curl play an important role in determining what hairstyles are practical for each person.

Because of the many factors that must be considered in selecting an appropriate hairstyle, consultation with an experienced beautician or stylist often helps. Consultation after cosmetic facial surgery is often especially rewarding as the new appearance is often enhanced and dramatized by selecting a different hairstyle.

Cosmetology and hairstyling have become specialized areas and women who have cosmetic facial surgery should be aware of the value of these techniques in enhancing appearance. Several books are available for those who want further information about this area.

Index